INTRODUCTION TO FLEXIBLE BRONCHOSCOPY

TRAINING MANUAL

SECOND EDITION

HENRI G COLT M.D. FAWM, FCCP

BRONCHOSCOPY INTERNATIONAL

THE BRONCHOSCOPY EDUCATION PROJECT SERIES

rake press

THE BRONCHOSCOPY EDUCATION PROJECT SERIES

SECOND EDITION

Henri G. Colt MD, FAWM, FCCP

This Second Edition of **The Bronchoscopy Education Project Series** of training manuals constitutes part of the highly regarded Bronchoscopy Education Project. These training manuals provide a broad perspective on the art, knowledge, science, and technical skills that must be acquired in order to be a competent bronchoscopist. They are written for bronchoscopy educators and all those who wish to improve upon their ability to teach and mentor bronchoscopists regardless of specialty. Of course, readers are encouraged to also study, *The Essential Bronchoscopist© Series* of learning materials and to participate in our many Faculty Development (train-the-Trainer) programs conducted all over the world in collaboration with many national bronchology and interventional associations.

Each **Training Manual** incorporates theories and instructional modalities as part of our competency-oriented training and mastery learning philosophies. Educational modalities are learner-centric, always emphasizing that the end result must be patient-driven.

Each volume in the series pertains to a different aspect of bronchoscopic practice. The overall structure of each volume, however, is similar, containing examples of on-site course agendas, a summary of reading materials, selected references, a description of step-by-step technical skill instruction, simulation workshop scenarios, patient-based practical approach exercises, validated assessment tools to monitor progress along the learning curve, and a series of checklists designed to enhance patient, operator, and equipment safety. Patients must no longer suffer the burden of physician learning.

Readers are encouraged to download additional materials from our website (www.bronchoscopy.org) and view instructional videos from the BronchOrg YouTube channel and other sources as well as attend regional seminars and participate in apprentice-like training experiences. With your help and the support of national organizations and associations such as the *World Association for Bronchology and Interventional Pulmonology*, **The Bronchoscopy Education Project** can help bring uniformity to medical procedural training for years to come.

Training Manuals

- INTRODUCTION TO FLEXIBLE BRONCHOSCOPY
- ENDOBRONCHIAL ULTRASOUND AND EBUS-GUIDED TBNA
- LEARNING AND TEACHING BRONCHOSCOPY

BRONCHOSCOPY INTERNATIONAL

Sponsored by Bronchoscopy International, Laguna Beach, CA 92651

Colt Henri G

Introduction to Flexible Bronchoscopy Training Manual
Bronchoscopy Education Project Series of Training Manuals

ISBN 978-0-9848347-0-9

1. Introduction to Flexible bronchoscopy

1. Colt HG, 1956-

Publisher Rake Press
Laguna Beach, CA

Manufactured in the United States of America

1 2 3 4 5 6 7 8 9 10

rake press

THE BRONCHOSCOPY EDUCATION PROJECT SERIES

INTRODUCTION TO FLEXIBLE BRONCHOSCOPY

TRAINING MANUAL

SECOND EDITION

HENRI G COLT MD, FAWM, FCCP

BRONCHOSCOPY INTERNATIONAL

With contributions from Drs S. Murgu, E. Edell, S. Quadrelli, and M. Davoudi, and J. Williamson.

Notice: Knowledge changes. We have done our best to assure references to procedures, medications, and techniques are correct and compatible with standards of practice at the time of publication. We are proud that Checklists, Assessment tools, and Bronchoscopy Step-by-Step instructional methods are commonly used around the world. Future editions may include modifications based on user feedback and new information. Any doctor, patient, or hospital names used in simulation/learning scenarios in this manual are fictitious.

Distributed by Bronchoscopy International*, The World Association for Bronchology and Interventional Pulmonology, and national bronchology and interventional pulmonology societies.

rake press

Printed in the United States

* Bronchoscopy International Foundation for the Advancement of Medicine; a 501c3 Non-Profit Foundation Registry # 33-0593357

ACKNOWLEDGMENTS

This Bronchoscopy Education Project training manual could not have been written without the help and advice of numerous colleagues from around the world who enthusiastically use the training modalities described herein. These regional champions are changing the paradigm of procedure-related learning to the great benefit of our patients and society. Their confidence in the process is particularly inspiring in the face of resistance from established practitioners who advocate a more conventional manner of instruction. Of course, my thanks also to patients everywhere who without questions have until recently suffered the burden of procedure-related training at the hands of health care professionals who learn solely by doing.

ABOUT THE AUTHOR

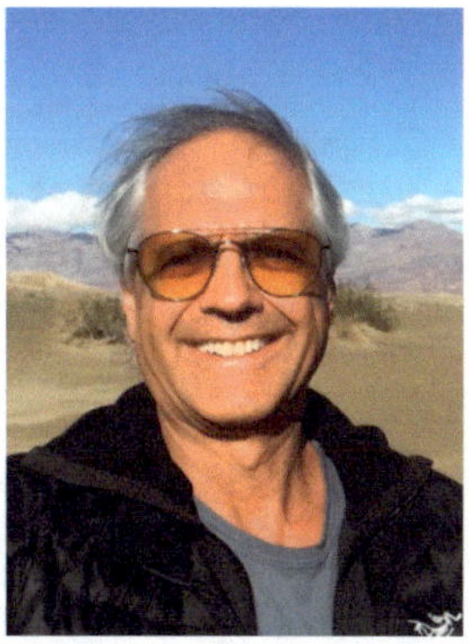

HENRI COLT is an award-winning medical educator, ethicist and philosophical practitioner. In addition to authoring scientific papers and several medical textbooks, he is the author/editor of the popular *The Picture of Health: Medical Ethics and the Movies* (Oxford University Press) and nonfiction works such as *Modigliani: Art & illness.* His *Essential Bronchoscopist* series of books and medical training tools have been translated into 14 languages. His *Bronchoscopy and Central Airway Disorders: A Patient-centered Approach* (Elsevier press) with coauthor Professor Septimiu Murgu is a textbook standard for Interventional pulmonologists and airway specialists around the world.

Dr. Colt is University of California Emeritus Professor of Pulmonary and Critical Care Medicine. When he is not traveling, writing or teaching, he is dancing tango or climbing mountains in far away places.

Funding statement

Funding for The Bronchoscopy Education Project Series is a result of philanthropic endeavors
No corporate support was either solicited or received for this work.

Bronchoscopy International® and The Essential Bronchoscopist® are official trademarks.

Bronchoscopy International is a transnational group of volunteers working under the auspices of The Foundation for the Advancement of Medicine, a 501-C3 non-profit organization registered in San Diego, CA, USA (Registry # 33-0593357).

Bronchoscopy Education Project Disclaimer

Confidentiality of data potentially relating to individual patients has been respected. We strive to honor or exceed any legal requirements of medical/health information privacy as they apply to the United States and to the state of California.

Images and case descriptions provided here-in, therefore, are not intended for the diagnosis of any specific patient. Any information found on the website or in this text should not be used as a substitute for medical care.

The authors disclaim liability, injury, or damage incurred as a consequence from the use of information. Reference to websites, instruments, or equipment portrayed in this material is not of commercial nature, nor does the inclusion imply endorsement.

Should documents or images from this material be copied for personal use, we request that materials remain unedited and unmodified unless for teaching purposes, that no fee be charged for copies or access to the information, that copyright notices and disclaimers remain attached, and that credit be given to The Bronchoscopy Education Project (suggested format Bronchoscopy International® www.bronchoscopy.org).

rake press

Table of Contents

WELCOME
to the
Bronchoscopy Education Project

This collection of competency-oriented tools and materials was designed with a philosophy of mastery training in mind. Competency is the minimum threshold acceptable for medical procedural practice. Bronchoscopy International is a collegial group of expert bronchoscopist-educators devoted to teaching using a paradigm in which patients never suffer the burden of procedure-related learning. While the learner-centric structure of the project targets bronchoscopy, it is readily applied to other procedural areas of medical training.

Part I of **The Bronchoscopy Education Project** is an **Introduction to Flexible Bronchoscopy©.** This competency program addresses bronchoscopy inspection, lavage, brushing and endobronchial biopsy, transbronchial lung biopsy and conventional transbronchial needle aspiration. This training manual can be used with **The Essential Bronchoscopist©** series of books. It combines the science of bronchoscopy with technical skill instruction, validated assessment tools to measure and document performance, simulation scenarios, patient-centered practical approach exercises, and checklists to enhance patient, operator and equipment safety. Learners may wish to begin by reading **The Essential Flexible Bronchoscopist©**, which is a compilation of 180 question/answer sets pertaining to flexible bronchoscopy.

Materials from the Bronchoscopy Education Project can be incorporated in whole or in part into training programs. Other learning and teaching materials are available at our website, www.bronchoscopy.org. Welcome to the exciting world of Bronchoscopy Education. We look forward to your comments as you use these materials.

Henri Colt M.D

Henri Colt MD., FAWM, FCCP
henricolt@Bronchoscopy.org

The Shifting Paradigm of Bronchoscopy Education

Halstedt's model of graduate medical education based on a see one, do one, teach one paradigm implemented in the last century has been the traditional method of acquired learning during medical apprenticeship. Its relevance has come into question because this educational model is adversely affected by constraints of training for a fixed period of time, the presumed need to assimilate material through formal didactic and on-site teachings, a lack of alternatives to learning on patients, a tendency towards variability[1,2], and a presumption that learning curves are climbed by performing a minimum number of procedures while assuming an escalating number of responsibilities during training. In the absence of competency-oriented examinations, currently written exams and numbers requirements for procedures still provide some objective criteria on which to base competency[3].

The paradigm shift in bronchoscopy education has now occurred[4]. It is simply a matter of time and education that teachers and mentors all over the world implement new educational programs and methodologies. The diversity of medical practice and training is now recognized, and already accounts for changing constructs of training curricula[5]. Time and cost restraints prompt physicians to find ways with which to incorporate teaching and procedure-related training into a more effective and efficient clinical practice (Figure 1, abstracted from reference 4). Teaching is increasingly separated from clinical service responsibilities, and educators are using competency-oriented tools rather than subjective assessments and "observed experience" to enhance training. Information is increasingly accessible through social media and electronic media libraries. Literature searches of peer reviewed journals and other publications are at the students' fingertips.

Furthermore, universities and professional societies provide web-based instruction and continued medical education so learners can study materials at their own pace and according to their own busy schedules. Flipped classroom techniques are being used to improve and workshop one-on-one practical performance sessions, and the proven value of inanimate model and computer-based simulation, in addition to the recognized effectiveness of patient surrogates, problem-based learning, and practice-based interactive sessions render experiential learning based solely on patient encounters increasingly obsolete. Finally, has become evident that neither patients nor their novice physicians should be submitted to the potentially unethical practice of learning by doing, especially early in the course of training.

In the following paragraphs we describe several elements of a bronchoscopy educational program based on the premise that patients not bear the burden of procedure-related training. While we focus on the art and practice of flexible bronchoscopy, we propose that similar curricular structure are applicable to all fields of procedural medical practice. A social mandate for effective, efficient, safe, and ethically responsible clinical care warrants that we reassess older educational methodologies, and that we incorporate new techniques into the learning process. These techniques can often be individualized according to a learner's needs, and may enhance an accelerated climb of a procedural learning curve, assist in imparting knowledge to learners outside of the patient practice setting, avoid many of the shortcomings of existing and well-recognized variations in medical training, and allow the design of a more structured, uniform competency-oriented curriculum that can be individually tailored to fill the needs of diverse practices, cultures, and medical environments[6].

In general, procedure-based education requires factual knowledge, technical skill, experience, and a recognition of the effect of patient-procedural interactions on personal affectivity[i]. *Knowledge* generally refers to the acquisition of information required by a physician to make a medical decision. In this regard, cognitive knowledge refers to studies of cognitive processes such as perception, comprehension, decision-making and problem-solving that affect the decision-making process, whereas medical reasoning might apply to the acquisition of a series of skills that enable a clinical decision[ii].

Assessments are often used to identify what and how much learners are learning, how well they are progressing in their acquisition of knowledge and skills, their position on the learning curve, and to help identify the strengths and weaknesses of a curriculum. A combination of low and high-stakes testing might be used to provide opportunities for bidirectional feedback, need for remedial intervention, establish criteria for competency or modify certain elements of curricular structure if learners' needs are not being sufficiently addressed[7]. High-stakes assessments usually entail a pass-fail threshold with significant consequences for the learner, whereas low-stakes assessments are often performed as part of a curriculum to judge progress in the acquisition of knowledge or skill. A competency-based educational curriculum, therefore, must include elements that are teachable, learnable and measurable. Hence, *competence* is defined as the verifiable assimilation of a specific set of knowledge, skills, behaviors, attitudes, and educational experiences required of trainees to complete such graduate medical education programs[8,9,10,11].

The bronchoscopy-related literature supports the paradigm shift whereby patients will no longer bear the burden of procedure-related training. In a review of several papers pertaining to the use of simulation for bronchoscopy education[12], simulation was demonstrated to help learners improve procedural efficiency and economy of movement, thoroughness and accuracy of airway examination, and incidence of airway wall trauma. Both lo- and hi-fidelity simulation have been shown to enhance physician competency in procedural skills, while saving time and accelerating a learner's ascent of the learning curve. Hi-fidelity simulation platforms using three-dimensional virtual anatomy and force feedback technology can be used to learn bronchoscopic inspection, biopsy, brushing, conventional transbronchial needle aspiration and convex-probe endobronchial ultrasound-guided-TBNA, although less expensive, lo-fidelity models comprised of molded silicone or excised animal airways, are also very effective[13,14,15,16,17]. In the last ten years, results from numerous studies show the many benefits of simulation-based training.

In addition to increasing learner satisfaction and interest, simulated environments and structured curricular learning create opportunities where the uniformization of information is enhanced, tasks can be practiced repeatedly, risks to patients are eliminated, and training scenarios can be tailored to individual

---

[i] How one perceives the experience and responds to situations from an emotional, psychological and behavioral perspective. This is different from experiential learning, which, for example, might entail one's accumulation of knowledge based on a series of similar cases.

[ii] For example, the knowledge of and ability to apply clinical pathways or algorithms, and justify one's diversion from an algorithmic pathway in certain circumstances.

learners' needs. Procedural skills acquired through practice on simulators are considered transferable to the clinical setting (Figure 2), and objective assessments performed at time of training helps identify errors and provides opportunities for repeated, focused practice without exposing patients to the discomfort of unnecessarily prolonged procedures. Reading assignments should probably be mandatory to assure compliance[18], and validated assessment tools can be incorporated into learning curricula to help identify acquisition of knowledge and skills[19], as well as to study the effectiveness of a learning program[iii].

In an attempt to provide a curriculum that might be widely available and broadly applicable in diverse medical cultures and practice environments, a six-part program was designed to be accessed, in part, via the Internet, but also incorporated in whole or in part into continued medical education postgraduate seminars or formal institution-based training programs. This program includes reading material, a growing pictorial and video atlas, a step-by-step exercise-based technique for learning bronchoscopic inspection, a series of didactic and interactive lectures pertaining to the art and science of bronchoscopy, an assortment of patient-centered practical approach exercises to assist with acquiring the knowledge and skills required for appropriate procedure-related medical decision-making, and a group of validated assessment and self-assessment tools[iv]. Many of these materials are available on the Bronchoscopy International website (www.Bronchoscopy.org)[v]. Instructional videos are accessible on the website as well as directly on the Bronchoscopy International You Tube and Facebook pages.

In order to further disseminate and eventually study the impact of these methodologies from an educational research perspective, the curriculum has been incorporated into the **Bronchoscopy Education Project**. The purpose of this project is to provide educators, training program directors, and bronchoscopists in practice or in-training with competency-oriented tools and materials that can be used to assess progression along the learning curve from novice to competent practitioner. The uniform curriculum is built on a template that includes course schedules, informational content[20], checklists[vi], validated assessment tools, description and use of training models, simulation scenarios, patient-centered practical approach exercises, and a series of didactic and interactive lectures[21].

The BEP has been officially endorsed by numerous national bronchology and interventional pulmonology organizations, as well as by the AABIP, EABIP, WABIP, and the ASER[vii]. Some of the original practical investigations of several elements from this curriculum were undertaken with the help of the Argentine Association for Bronchology and Esophagology and The Singapore Thoracic Society. Faculty development programs are ongoing to help educators assimilate assorted techniques, implement educational methodologies,

---

[iii] Such as one that includes a one or two-day program of didactic lectures, hands-on learning, and interactive case-based scenarios. Class-average normalized gain (in addition to the calculation of absolute and relative gain) can be particularly helpful in this regard. (g) is defined as the average actual gain divided by the maximum possible gain (see Colt HG, et al., Surg Endosc 2011;25:207-216, available from the authors on request)

[iv] For example, The Essential Bronchoscopist© now translated into nine languages, the EBUS Bronchoscopist©, BronchAtlas™, the Art of Bronchoscopy©, Bronchoscopy Step-by-Step©, Practical Approach to Procedural Decision-Making, and Bronchoscopy Assessment Tools© (Bronchoscopy Skills and Tasks© [BSTAT], Bronchoscopy Self- Assessment Tool [BSAT], and Endobronchial Ultrasound Skills and Tasks© [EBUS-STAT].

[v] Bronchoscopy International is a no hierarchal group of motivated bronchoscopy educators serving as an integrated part of the 501-C3 non-profit Foundation for the Advancement of Medicine.

[vi] Examples of Checklists include Fluoroscopy, Informed Consent, Procedural pause, Moderate sedation, Practical approach, Proctored flexible bronchoscopy, and Program completion.

[vii] Abbreviations for American Association for Bronchology and Interventional Pulmonology, European Association for Bronchology and Interventional Pulmonology, World Association for Bronchology and Interventional Pulmonology, Asociaccion Sudamericana Endoscopia Respiratoria

master the application of the various assessment tools, practice their delivery of didactic lectures, and facilitate of interactive sessions. Programs provide opportunities for self-assessment, acquisition of debriefing skills and 360-degree feedback to enhance teaching skills[22,23]. These programs are made available through the generous support and assistance of international volunteer faculty, training institutions, and national or international societies, with the addition of material support for hands-on learning stations provided from equipment manufacturers and the World Association for Bronchology and Interventional Pulmonology.

We believe interventional pulmonary procedures such as bronchoscopy are performed more competently by bronchoscopists who possess a uniform foundation of theoretic knowledge and standardized skill. The uniformization of educational content and process has the potential to facilitate social interactions, knowledge transfer, and equality of care regardless of one's medical practice environment. The paradigm shift in bronchoscopy education, however, should not be taken lightly. Curricular content needs to be regularly revised and new assessment tools will require validation in specific target settings. Philosophies of competency-oriented training and mastery learning are not easily adopted without significant effort, and more research is warranted to assess their effectiveness.

Figure 1: Educational methodologies. From, Colt HG and Williamson J Respirology. 2020 25(9):997-1007.

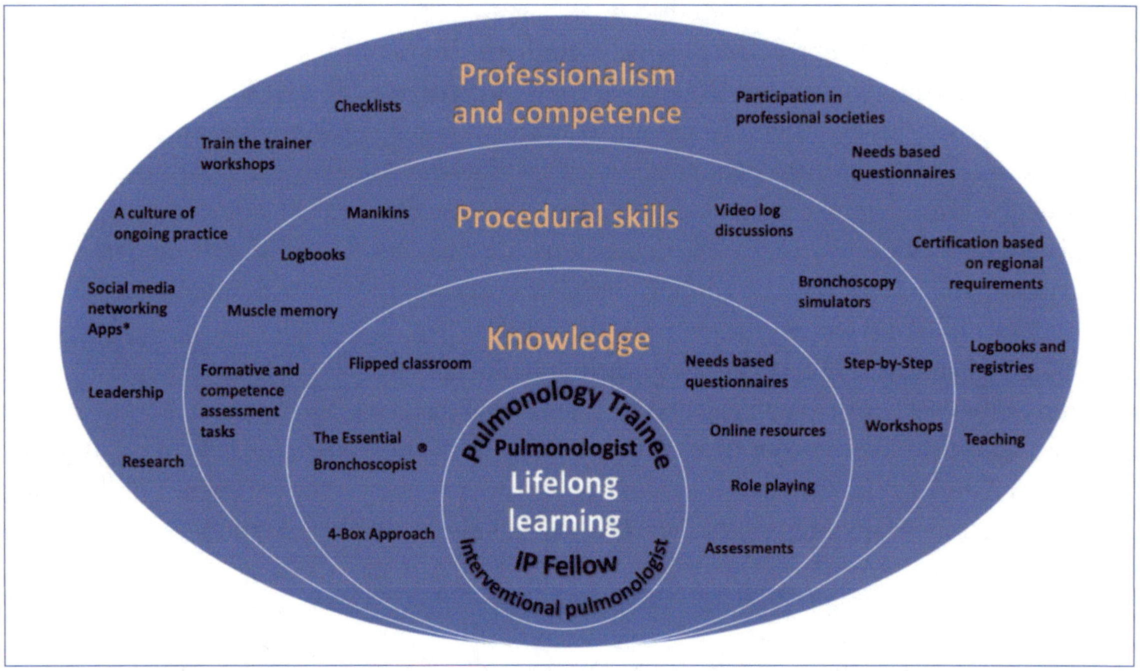

Figure 2: Examples of inanimate and computer-based simulation models for learning flexible bronchoscopy.

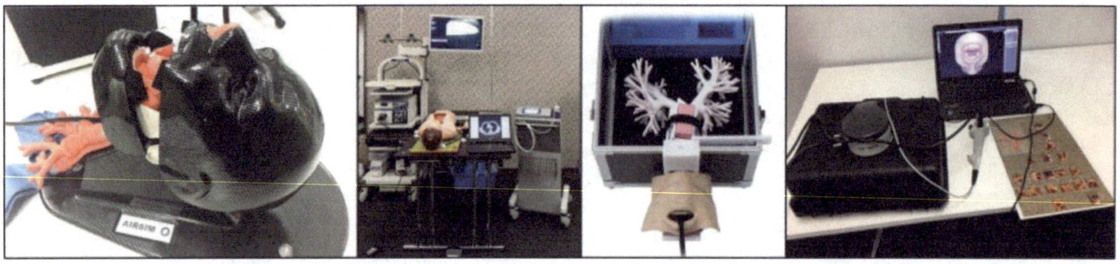

References

1. Pastis N, Silvestri, G et al. ACCP interventional chest diagnostic procedures network steering committee. Variation in training for interventional pulmonary procedures among US pulmonary critical care fellowships, a survey of Fellowship directors. Chest. 2005; 127:1614 – 1621.
2. Pyng L, Loo CM, Jagadesan R, Colt HG. Survey of bronchoscopy practice in Singapore. J Bronchol 2008;15(4):215-220.
3. Torrington KG. Bronchoscopy training and competency: How many are enough? Chest 1999;118:572-573.
4. Colt HG, Williamson JP. Training in interventional pulmonology: What we have learned and a way forward. Respirology. 2020 Sep;25(9):997-1007. doi: 10.1111/resp.13846. Epub 2020 May 26. PMID: 32453479.
5. Haponik EF, Russell GB, Beamis JF, et al. Bronchoscopy training: Current fellows, experiences, and some concerns for the future. Chest. 2000; 118:572 – 573.
6. Long DM. Competency based residency training: the next advance in graduate medical education. Academic Medicine 2000;75(12):1178-1183.
7. Quadrelli S, Galíndez F, Davoudi M Colt HG. Reliability of a 25 item *low stakes* multiple choice assessment of bronchoscopic knowledge. Chest 2009;135:315-321.
8. Marinopoulos SS, Baumann MH. Methods and definitions of terms: effectiveness of continuing medical education: American College of Chest Physicians evidence-based educational guidelines. Chest 2009;135:17S–28S.
9. Patel VL, Aroca JF, and Zhang J. Thinking, and reasoning in medicine. In The Cambridge handbook of thinking and reasoning. KJ Holyoake & Morrison RG Editors. University Press, Cambridge UK 2005.
10. High stakes testing "http://en.wikipedia.org/wiki/High-stakes_testing". Retrieved on March 20, 2008.
11. Miller GE. The assessment of clinical skills, competence and performance. Academic medicine 1990;65 (9 supplements): S63–7.
12. Davoudi M, Colt HG. Bronchoscopy simulation: a brief review. Adv Health Sci Educ 2009;14:287-296.
13. Davoudi M, Wahidi MM, Rohani NZ, Colt HG. Comparative effectiveness of low and high-fidelity bronchoscopy simulation for training in conventional transbronchial needle aspiration and user preferences. Respiration 2010;80:327-334.
14. Ost D, DeRosiers A, Britt EJ, et al. Assessment of a bronchoscopy simulator. Am J Respir Crit Care Med 2001;164(12):2248-55.
15. Crawford SW and Colt HG. Virtual reality and written assessments are of potential value to determine knowledge and skill in flexible bronchoscopy. Respiration 2004; 71:269 – 275.
16. Colt HG, Crawford, SW., Galbraith O. Virtual reality bronchoscopy simulation: A revolution in procedural training. Chest 2001; 120(4):1333–1339.
17. Goldberg R, Colt HG, Davoudi M, Cherisson L. Realistic and affordable lo-fidelity model for learning transbronchial needle aspiration. Surg Endosc;2009 Sep; 23(9): 2047-52.
18. Wahidi MM, Silvestri GA, Coakley RD, Ferguson JS, Shepherd RW, Moses L, Conforti J, Que L, Anstrom KJ, McGuire F, Colt H, Downie GH. A prospective multi-center study of competency metrics and educational interventions in the learning of bronchoscopy among starting pulmonary fellows. Chest 2010;137(5):1040-1049.
19. Davoudi M, Osann K, and Colt HG. Validation of two instruments to assess technical bronchoscopy skill using virtual reality simulation. Respiration 2008;76:92-101.
20. Davoudi M, Quadrelli S, Osann K, and Colt HG. A competency-based test of bronchoscopic knowledge using the Essential Bronchoscopist: an initial concept study. Respirology 2008;13:736-743.
21. Colt HG, Davoudi M, Murgu S, and Rohani NZ. Measuring learning gain during a one-day introductory bronchoscopy course. Surg Endoscopy 2010;25:207-216.
22. Rudolph JW, Simon R, Dufresne RL, et al. There's no such thing as nonjudgemental debriefing. A theory and method for debriefing with good judgement. Simulation in Healthcare 2006;1:49-55.
23. Goldsmith M and Underhill B. 2001. Multisource feedback for executive development. In D. Bracken, C Timmreck and A. Church (eds). The handbook of multi-source feedback, pp 275-288. Jossey-Bass: San Francisco.

Training in Interventional Pulmonology: New ways Forward

Extracted in part from: Colt HG, Williamson JP. Training in interventional pulmonology: What we have learned and a way forward. Respirology. 2020 Sep; 25(9):997-1007. doi: 10.1111/resp.13846. Epub 2020 May 26. PMID: 32453479.

Until recently, training strategies for Interventional pulmonology (IP) were intrinsically linked to the see one, do one, teach one apprentice-style model traditionally used for centuries in medical education. Teaching methodologies were patriarchal in nature, often reflecting power differentials between teacher and learner, as well as hierarchal structures and the idea that it is was permissible to use patients as a basis for learning.

Thankfully, times are changing. According to data from the Association of American Medical Colleges, medical schools in the United States are increasingly diverse, and women now make up more than 50% of classes, a trend also found in many other countries[1]. Furthermore, increased familiarity with social media and the internet makes sharing information and experience instantaneous. New educational paradigms focused on the democratization of knowledge encourage access to these technologies, as well as to using inanimate models and computer-based simulation rather than patients to practice and perfect procedural skills. These methods allow independent learning with a focus on objective measures of competence using specifically-designed assessment tools that are now accepted, not only for measuring technical skills, but also for demonstrating skills with problem-solving, differential diagnosis, informed consent and other components of the medical encounter.

Radical, disruptive, and transformative changes do not occur without challenges. People and institutions are reluctant to abandon traditional ways of thinking and slow to adapt to new paradigms. This natural resistance, coupled with the accelerating speed of technological evolution and conflicts faced in teaching environments where optimal patient care must be balanced with cost concerns, time-efficiency, expectations for quality, safety, and accountability, as well as with an instructor's goal to impart knowledge and the trainee's desire to master skills essential to their careers, provides a situational background that is common to many countries.

Indeed, the nature of interventional pulmonology suggests that training programs should provide learners with a broad exposure to more than just technical skills. Opportunities to assess the acquisition of many forms of knowledge, including those needed to nurture humanistic qualities and medical expertise are also desirable. Of course, there is a minimum requirement for practitioners is to dedicate time and energy to learning bronchoscopy and other interventional procedures under the guidance of experts. The increasing number of possible interventions, in addition to decreased durations of hospitalizations, a limited source of patients, overwhelming amounts of information and procedure-related technologies, and rising health care costs makes it essential for anyone learning procedures to master what some might call basic, but which I prefer calling the 'foundations' of bronchoscopic practice. This includes technical skills, and everything linked to the multidisciplinary and multidimensional patient care environment in which informed patients participate actively in management decisions.

Traditionally, numbers of procedures were a metric upon which attaining competency was based. However, a purely numbers-based training program does not equate to competency, and is insufficient on its own[2,3]. Numbers represent hands-on experience in the patient-care setting, but without oversight and structured feedback by trained teachers/mentors, they are of little value. Oversight might take the form of direct observation, distance-monitoring in real-time, or post-hoc reviews of recorded case videos. Feedback through two-way instructor-learner communication based on the use of objective measures or checklists will help improve knowledge and technical skills for both observed as well as hypothetical procedure-related issues.

We believe, therefore, that every hospital department should provide bronchoscopists with manikins or affordable and ideally, free access to simulation so they and their teams can maintain and improve their skills through repetitive, task-driven practice[4,5]. I am constantly puzzled as to why so many university hospitals around the world still refuse to commit small amounts of money to purchase such models so their faculty and trainees might improve and maintain their skills without causing undue suffering or prolonged procedures in patients.

Of course, there is still debate regarding how assessment tools might serve as measures of competency. Score-based assessments if conducted serially, can identify weaknesses to be remedied by individualized training, thus establishing a minimum standard of competency that is potentially confirmed using a high-stakes examination with cut-off scores or pass/fail criteria. This approach helps assure patient safety as well as the ethical and appropriate performance of a particular procedure often required by hospital accreditation committees in credentialing individual practitioners. Other assessments might include multiple-choice style examinations to document learner participation in a predefined number of workshops, charting observations of a learner's behavior during interactive small-group exercises, mandating completion of a specified duration of apprentice-style training, and reviewing procedure-related experience with videos and procedural logbooks.[6,7,8]

Given the above, we caution against learning by doing. Instead, we suggest learners participate in structured, multidimensional educational programs, albeit with a caveat: All learners have varying levels of experience. Some are already competent proceduralists whilst others are beginners, and of course, one may even be an expert in one procedure, yet have novice or intermediate abilities in another. Allowing for individualization and acknowledging that all learners learn differently, adds value to a learner-centric educational approach. Furthermore, training programs should nurture ethical behaviors and scientific curiosity through active participation and growing responsibilities in multidisciplinary interdepartmental meetings, research projects, teaching of more junior colleagues, and by giving an increased place to arguably "soft medicine" subjects alongside science and technology at national conferences and workshops. The role of mentoring is undeniable, and even decision-making and communication skills can be learned. The purpose of our Train-the Trainers programs has been to help teach teachers how to teach. Bronchoscopy

International has conducted more than forty such programs all over the world, and they are received with great enthusiasm, resulting also in a number of certified and master instructors who are able to carry on the mission in their own countries and regions.

We believe that dedicated teaching moments are preferable to teaching on-the-job during clinical/service rounds because most learners have facts, figures, and much of the published literature at their fingertips using mobile devices. In regards to structured curricula and implementing a more uniform model for IP education, the United States now has several 12 to 24-month programs with centralized application processes, published standards for program curricula, and exit examinations. Italy has an extensive curriculum for IP training, including a Master's program through the University of Florence, and, more recently Ancona, providing a link between an academic university-based program for didactic and course-oriented studies with affiliated teaching hospitals to provide the necessary hands-on procedural experience. The European Respiratory Society has an IP accreditation program built around EBUS, and a professional certification program covering theory, online self-directed modules, quizzes, webcasts, course and live case attendance, hands-on simulation training, and submission of a logbook and video cases for review, The Thoracic Society of Australia and New Zealand instituted regional training seminars, procedural log reviews, and encourages using a variety of validated assessment tools while actively building a cadre of Bronchoscopy International® certified and master instructors. In Argentina, a one-year certification program in bronchoscopy includes a multidimensional curriculum, objective measures of knowledge and technical skill, procedural log reviews, multiple opportunities for targeted practice using airway models and manikins, and supervised hands-on training. Similar programs are being designed elsewhere in South America, Romania, Serbia, India, Bangladesh, Malaysia, Indonesia, and Algeria.[9,10,11,12,13]

Technical skills require *muscle memory*. Research shows that neural pathways can be formed, and habits developed by combining many small tasks learned incrementally before combining them into more complex procedures. These skills can be practiced and perfected using inanimate models and computer-based simulation[14,15]. This is similar to the way one learns to play a musical instrument or swing a golf club. We believe that training programs that allow individualization through the identification of strengths and weaknesses using such objective measures also help identify a minimum standard of competency that might be universally accepted regardless of one's country or region of practice. The "Step by Step" method of bronchoscopy training is one example of gradual acquisition of muscle memory whereby trainees acquire skills by deconstructing a complex procedure into numbered steps that are taught individually and combined gradually until the entire procedure is performed[16].

In a multidimensional, structured learning environment, the acquisition of psychomotor skills is ideally accompanied by the acquisition of cognitive (theoretical, metacognitive, and factual), affective (growth in how feelings and emotions might affect decision-making), and experiential (as opposed to a-priori) knowledge. This is accomplished through minor alterations to the apprenticeship-style model and lends credence to the use of small group, case-based instruction using real or fabricated case scenarios. We have incorporated role-playing exercises into our Train-the-Trainer programs with great success and participation satisfaction. Role-playing exercises are also beneficial and popular for practicing communication skills. Independent learning in our programs is encouraged using social media platforms and programs designed for mobile devices. Online resources include Bronchoscopy International® (www.Bronchoscopy.org); Uptodate® in Pulmonary Medicine; Panminerva Medica's comprehensive articles on training needs, competency requirements, and state-of-the-art reviews; online bronchoscopy simulation and YouTube instructional videos, Facebook such as www.facebook.com/groups/pleural.hub/; and dozens of national Bronchology groups representing more than 5000 physicians communicating in real-time using WhatsApp. This forum was of incredible value during the recent SARS-CoV-2 pandemic.

Because time with an instructor is precious, a Flipped Classroom model is also attractive[17]. This differs from a traditional classroom model because materials are usually provided before on-site learning, and students are asked to consider, reflect, and explore content often as homework or during interactive small group sessions. The teacher's role changes from classroom-based lecturer to attentive coach and supportive facilitator. Such an approach lends itself well to problem-based learning methods such as those used in our 4-Box Practical Approach exercises[18].

Hospital-based teaching is usually not done in a formal setting, and frequently, face to face contact between student and teacher occurs at the patient's bedside, in clinical consultation rooms, or the procedure suite. These moments provide priceless opportunities to impart and reinforce knowledge, involve the trainee in care discussions and management plans, provide career advice, and identify a learner's needs. We suggest adding a dedicated moment for teaching, rather than teaching on-the-run, to help distinguish between clinical service (doing the work, providing patient care) and education (where teachers and learners work together to enhance each other's knowledge, skill, and experience).

In regards to using simulation for bronchoscopy training, the existence of commercially available airway manikins and newer disposable bronchoscopes provides a relatively low-cost alternative whilst maintaining a remarkable degree of anatomical realism with a true to life sense of bronchoscope handling. Manikins are often preferable to computer-based simulation for learning to remove foreign bodies, sample endobronchial masses, and suction airway secretions or blood. A single-use disposable bronchoscope costing a few hundred dollars can be reserved for educational purposes and used hundreds of times coupled with an inexpensive display panel[19,20]. A 3D printed airway cast, being a less expensive, custom-made device, may provide even more realism than many expensive commercial units[21].

Results from simulation studies show a demonstrable increase in the acquisition of dexterity skills, improvements in the speed of airway inspection, numbers of segments visualized, reduced airway wall collisions and faster performance on the learning curve early in training; as few as 20 simulated procedures is significantly associated with increased acquisition of bronchoscopy skills on validated assessment tasks. Studies also show superior performance in patients for trainees who learned initially on a simulator compared to those who did not, a finding that is consistent with results from simulator studies in other subspecialties. Laptop-sized models are also available and can be carried to courses.[22,23,24,25,26,27]

If competency is defined as a combination of observable and measurable skills, knowledge, and behaviors, it follows that an assessment strategy using a collection of specific tools and methodologies is required. Among others, these encompass objective forms for measuring, monitoring, and reviewing one's technical skill and knowledge, as well as one's ability to plan a procedure, obtain results similar to those of one's peers, and respond appropriately to procedure-related complications. As alluded to earlier, we also believe competency should be demonstrated in peri-procedural aspects of care such as the ability to obtain informed consent, deliver news of a diagnosis in a culturally sensitive and appropriate manner, communicate effectively with colleagues and patients, perform effectively as a team leader, and develop a satisfactory follow-up procedural plan. This should be accompanied with a greater knowledge and understanding of how medical ethics are applied to interventional pulmonology.

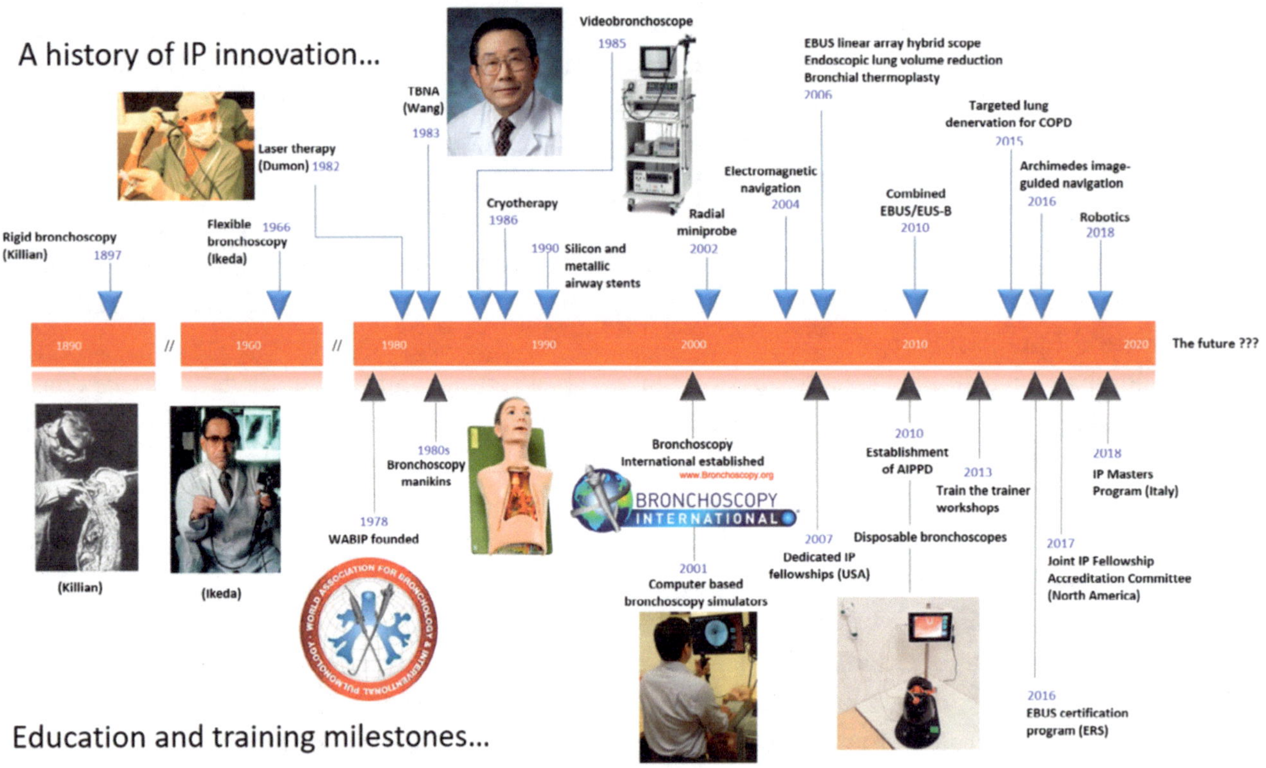

History of IP Innovation. From Colt HG, Williamson JP. Training in interventional pulmonology: What we have learned and a way forward. Respirology. 2020 Sep;25(9):997-1007

References

1. Colleges AoAM. 2018 Fall applicant and matriculant data tables. Association of American Medical Colleges; 2018 December 2018.
2. Wahidi MM, Silvestri G, Conforti J, et al. Assessment of pulmonary fellow acquisition of bronchoscopy skills. *Chest*. 2007;132(4):514C.
3. Downie G, Bowling M, Silvestri G, et al. The Multi-State Bronchoscopy Education Project: acquisition of cognitive skills. *Chest Journal*. 2007;132.
4. Voduc N, Dudek N, Parker CM, et al. Development and Validation of a Bronchoscopy Competence Assessment Tool in a Clinical Setting. *Ann Am Thorac Soc*. 2016;13(4):495-501.
5. Wahidi MM, Silvestri GA, Coakley RD, et al. A prospective multicenter study of competency metrics and educational interventions in the learning of bronchoscopy among new pulmonary fellows. *Chest*. 2010;137(5):1040-9.
6. Salamonsen MR, Bashirzadeh F, Ritchie AJ, et al. A new instrument to assess physician skill at chest tube insertion: the TUBE-iCOMPT. *Thorax*. 2015;70(2):186-8.
7. Dalal PG, Dalal GB, Pott L, et al. Learning curves of novice anesthesiology residents performing simulated fibreoptic upper airway endoscopy. *Can J Anaesth*. 2011;58(9):802-9.
8. Corbetta L, Arru LB, Mereu C, et al. Competence and training in interventional pulmonology. *Panminerva Med*. 2019;61(3):203-31.
9. Mullon JJ, Burkart KM, Silvestri G, et al. Interventional Pulmonology Fellowship Accreditation Standards: Executive Summary of the Multisociety Interventional Pulmonology Fellowship Accreditation Committee. *Chest*. 2017;151(5):1114-21.

10. Corbetta L, Patelli M. Executive Summary of Training and Competence Standards for the Interventional Pulmonology Master Program in Italy. *J Bronchology Interv Pulmonol.* 2018;25(1):6-8.
11. Williamson JP, Twaddell SH, Lee YCG, et al. Thoracic ultrasound recognition of competence: A position paper of the Thoracic Society of Australia and New Zealand. *Respirology*. 2017;22(2):405-8.
12. Miller GE. The assessment of clinical skills/competence/performance. *Acad Med.* 1990;65(9 Suppl):S63-7.
13. Farr A, Clementsen P, Herth F, et al Endobronchial ultrasound: launch of an ERS structured training programme. *Breathe*. 2016;12(3):217-20.
14. Davoudi M, Osann K, Colt HG. Validation of two instruments to assess technical bronchoscopic skill using virtual reality simulation. *Respiration*. 2008;76(1):92-101.
15. Ost D, Rosiers AD, Britt EJ, et ale. Assessment of a Bronchoscopy Simulator. *American Journal of Respiratory and Critical Care Medicine*. 2001;164(12):2248-55.
16. Bronchoscopy International [cited 2019 7-12-2019]. Available from: https://bronchoscopy.org/step-by-step.
17. Baker JW. The "Classroom Flip": Using Web course management tools to become the guide by the side. In: Chambers JA, editor. Selected papers from the 11th International Conference on College Teaching and Learning. Jacksonville, Florida: Florida Community College at Jacksonville; 2000. p. 9-17.
18. Colt HG and Murgu S. *Bronchoscopy and Central Airways Obstruction*: A Patient-Centered Approach. New York, Saunders 2012.
19. Baker PA, Weller JM, Baker MJ, et al. Evaluating the ORSIM(R) simulator for assessment of anaesthetists' skills in flexible bronchoscopy: aspects of validity and reliability. *Br J Anaesth*. 2016;117 Suppl 1:i87-i91.
20. Garner JL, Garner SD, Hardie RJ, et al. Evaluation of a re-useable bronchoscopy biosimulator with ventilated lungs. *ERJ Open Res*. 2019;5(2):00035-2019.
21. Pedersen TH, Gysin J, Wegmann A, et al. A randomised, controlled trial evaluating a low cost, 3D-printed bronchoscopy simulator. *Anaesthesia*. 2017;72(8):1005-9.
22. Blum MG, Powers TW, Sundaresan S. Bronchoscopy simulator effectively prepares junior residents to competently perform basic clinical bronchoscopy. *Ann Thorac Surg*. 2004;78(1):287-91; discussion -91.
23. Cook DA, Hatala R, Brydges R, et al. Technology-enhanced simulation for health professions education: a systematic review and meta-analysis. *Jama*. 2011;306(9):978-88.
24. Clay AS, Gold JA. Teaching with Simulation. In: Kritek PA, Richards JB, editors. Medical Education in Pulmonary, Critical Care, and Sleep Medicine: Advanced Concepts and Strategies. Cham: Springer International Publishing; 2019. p. 213-33.
25. Konge L, Arendrup H, von Buchwald C, et al. Using Performance in Multiple Simulated Scenarios to Assess Bronchoscopy Skills. *Respiration*. 2011;81(6):483-90.
26. Colt HG, Davoudi M, Murgu S, et al. Measuring learning gain during a one-day introductory bronchoscopy course. *Surg Endosc*. 2011;25(1):207-16.
27. Miller RJ, Mudambi L, Vial MR, et al. Evaluation of Appropriate Mediastinal Staging among Endobronchial Ultrasound Bronchoscopists. *Ann Am Thorac Soc*. 2017;14(7):1162-8.

****

Introduction to Flexible Bronchoscopy Program Learning Objectives

This program is designed for long-term use. Learners will acquire and improve on their skills during a lifetime of learning and practice. Practitioners may wish to enter this program in order to improve or supplement their knowledge and skills. Others will participate in this program as part of their subspecialty training.

The program was developed so that parts could be learned by participating in regional seminars. Other aspects of the program will require dedicated study and practice during the course of one's training.

By the end of this program, participants will have achieved the following objectives:

- Acquired cognitive knowledge of bronchoscopy and bronchoscopic practice as demonstrated by passing scores on all six modules of the Flexible Essential Bronchoscopist©.
- Acquired technical skill enabling the independent performance of diagnostic flexible bronchoscopy as demonstrated by passing scores on Bronchoscopy step-by-step, and proctored checklists.
- Acquired cognitive, technical, affective, and experiential knowledge and skills as required in case of consultation for flexible bronchoscopy as documented by passing scores on the patient-centered practical approach exercise checklist.
- Ability to describe and perform the major elements of informed consent, moderate sedation, fluoroscopy, procedural pause, and patient safety as demonstrated by 100% passing scores on each of the associated checklists.
- Ability to technically perform a diagnostic flexible bronchoscopy, use common nomenclature, and recognize abnormal mucosal and secretion changes as documented by passing scores using BSTAT and BSTAT-TBLB/TBNA, and on-line independent study of images in BronchAtlas® and Art of Bronchoscopy©.
- Acquired confidence performing diagnostic flexible bronchoscopy as documented using BSAT.

The Introduction to Flexible Bronchoscopy Curriculum

1. Welcome to the Bronchoscopy Education Project training materials
2. Examples of *Regional Introductory course* schedules with didactic lectures, interactive sessions and simulation-based hands-on workshops using a pre-test/post-test model to document cognitive knowledge and technical skill acquisition.
3. Overview of suggested reading assignments:
   - *The Essential Flexible Bronchoscopist©*, a six module, 186 question/answer study guide with learning objectives and module-specific post-tests.
   - *Moderate Sedation* Module with lecture, synopsis and associated checklist.
   - *Fluoroscopy* Module with lecture, synopsis and associated checklist.
4. *Bronchoscopy Step-by-Step* exercises, instructional videos and associated checklist.
5. Hands-on *simulation-based workshop scenarios* using role-playing, low and high-fidelity models and the following scenarios:
   - *Informed consent, Procedural pause, and Patient safety* (includes overview of universal, droplet, and airborne pathogens precautions).
   - *Flexible bronchoscopy inspection with BAL, biopsy and brushing.*
   - *Flexible bronchoscopy inspection with TBLB and/or TBNA*
6. A series of *observed real-patient scenarios* including:
   - *Informed consent, Procedural pause and Patient safety.*
   - *Flexible bronchoscopy inspection with BAL, biopsy* and *brushing.*
   - *Flexible bronchoscopy inspection with transbronchial lung biopsy and/or transbronchial needle aspiration.*
7. Interactive *Patient-centered Practical Approach to Procedural Decision-making* workshops
8. A *proctored real patient bronchoscopy* with competency checklist assessment.
9. A collection of *Bronchoscopy Assessment Tools* to monitor progress:
   - Bronchoscopy Skills and Tasks Assessment Tool (BSTAT)
   - BSTAT-TBLB & TBNA Assessment Tool
   - Bronchoscopy Self-Assessment Tool (BSAT)
   - The Essential Flexible Bronchoscopist post-tests and answers

10. An excerpt from the *Train-the-Trainers Manual* and course curriculum, including instructions on how to use this Introduction to Flexible Bronchoscopy Curriculum, Bronchoscopy Assessment Tools and Checklists.
11. A collection of *Checklists* to enhance patient, operator, and equipment safety:
    - Fluoroscopy checklist
    - Moderate sedation checklist
    - Informed consent checklist
    - Procedural pause and Patient safety checklist
    - Practical Approach checklist
    - Bronchoscopy step-by-step checklist
    - Proctored flexible bronchoscopy checklist
    - Program completion checklist
12. Congratulations

SECTION 1

Regional Courses

Regional Introduction to Flexible Bronchoscopy programs are comprised of didactic lectures, interactive sessions and simulation-based hands-on workshops, often using a pre-test/post-test model to document cognitive knowledge and technical skill acquisition.

USER INSTRUCTIONS:

Regional Introduction to Flexible Bronchoscopy Programs (IFP)

Learning bronchoscopy in the clinical setting promotes learner anxiety, forces patients to suffer the burden of medical procedure-related learning [1], and results in a highly variable learning experience [2]. Clinical responsibilities often interfere with reading of bronchoscopy-related material, and, in the absence of periodic assessments of bronchoscopy-related knowledge, trainees are unlikely to be compliant with educational endeavors they perceive as optional or reliant on individual motivation, especially if there are no pass/fail grading consequences [3]. The current subspecialty bronchoscopy learning environment is further rendered less-than-ideal for beginners because of concerns regarding patient safety, fiscal constraints, and an increasing impetus to document procedural competency [4-6].

Whilst not supplanting on-the-job training that occurs with subspecialty rotations, short postgraduate courses comprised of lectures and simulation-based hands-on instruction, have thus become a popular means towards enhancing procedure-related learning [7-9]. In accordance with continued medical education (CME) guidelines, these programs identify learner objectives and provide opportunities for feedback from students regarding the perceived quality of the course.

The purpose of regional courses is to provide standardized learning material to bronchoscopy trainees. By regionalizing the process, program directors can enlist participants from numerous regional programs, thereby reducing course-related expenditures pertaining to travel and lodging. Already, several courses have become highly popular in the Carolinas, Southern California, and Midwest. Other regional courses are occurring in the Asia, Latin America and Australia. During course participation, learners are exposed to uniform course material delivered using didactic lectures, interactive sessions, hands-on training using patient models, low-fidelity and high-fidelity simulation, debriefing exercises, and problem-based learning modules. Pre-test/post-test assessments help document knowledge and technical skill acquisition, thereby setting a new baseline for learners in subspecialty training.

It has long been recognized that assessment drives learning, and that rigorous assessment inspires learning, reinforces confidence, and reassures the public. Proving that course participation is responsible for learning gains is difficult. For example, demonstrating the short-term benefit of an educational intervention is controversial because of debates regarding the value of pre-test and post-test assessments, and because of the obvious difficulty constituting a control group to which studies of an educational intervention can be compared [10-13]. Studies of long-term retention are problematic because causality is subject to the effects of normal maturation and ongoing training history [14].

The true value of pre-test/post-test assessments has also been controversial because of the effects of many extraneous variables, which include the Hawthorne effect (knowing that one is being tested may affect the results), the halo effect (the human tendency to respond positively or negatively to an instructor), and the practice effect (of a pre-test on a subsequent post-test). In the context of procedure-based training, the calculation of various measures of learning gain, including class-average and single-student normalized gain provides an objective and informative means to document learner performance and demonstrate robustness of the educational intervention.

Patients should not suffer the burden of procedure-related learning. Participation in regional courses, using simulation-based deliberate practice to acquire technical skill, and documenting a rapid climb up the initially steep slope of the novice's learning curve should result in decreased patient suffering and improved procedure-related decision making. Diverse opinions regarding educational methodologies, curricular structure, and measures of effectiveness persist in regards to short one- or two-day programs [15-16]. Additional studies are needed to document effectiveness and to determine how regional courses might favorably impact patient outcomes.

Selected References

1. Silvestri GA. The evolution of bronchoscopy training. Respiration. 2008;76(1):92-101.
2. Haponik EF, Russell GB, Beamis JF, et al. Bronchoscopy training: current fellows' experiences and some concerns for the future. Chest. 2000 Sep;118(3):572-573.
3. Wahidi MM, Silvestri GA, Coakley RD, Ferguson JS, Shepherd RW, Moses L, Conforti J, Que L, Anstrom KJ, McGuire F, Colt H, Downie GH. A prospective multi-center study of competency metrics and educational interventions in the learning of bronchoscopy among starting pulmonary fellows. Chest 2010;137(5):1040-1049.
4. Reznick RK, MacRae H. Teaching Surgical Skills – Changes in the Wind. N Engl J Ned. 2006; 355:2664-2669.
5. Carraccio C, Englander R. Evaluating competence using a portfolio: a literature review and web-based application to the ACGME competencies. Teach Learn Med. 2004 Fall;16(4):381-387.
6. Carraccio C, Wolfsthal SD, Englander R, et al. Shifting Paradigms: From Flexner to Competencies. Academic Medicine. 2002;77(5):361-367.
7. Norman G. The American College of Chest Physicians evidence-based educational guidelines for continuing medical education interventions: a critical review of evidence-based educational guidelines. Chest. 2009;135(3):834-837.
8. Schijven MP, Schout BM, Dolmans VE, Hendrikx AJ, Broeders IA, Borel Rinkes IH. Perceptions of surgical specialists in general surgery, orthopaedic surgery, urology and gynaecology on teaching endoscopic surgery in The Netherlands. Surg Endosc. 2008;22(2):472-482.
9. Davis D, Bordage G, Moores LK, Bennett N, Marinopoulos SS, Mazmanian PE, Dorman T, McCrory D. The Science of Continuing Medical Education. Chest.2009;135:8S-16S.
10. Cronbach LJ, Furby L. How should we measure "change" or should we? Psychol. Bull 1970;74:68-80.
11. Hake, R.R. 2009. "Should We Measure Change? Yes!" <http://www.physics.indiana.edu/~hake>. And <http://www.physics.indiana.edu/~hake/MeasChangeS.pdf> (2.5 MB)
12. Melzer DE. Normalized learning gain: A key measure of student learning [Addendum to: Melzer DE. The relationship between mathematics preparation and conceptual learning gains in physics: A possible "hidden variable" in diagnostic pretest scores. Am J. Phys 2002;70:1259-1267. Online http://scitation.aip.org/getpdf/servlet/GetPDFServlet?filetype=pdf&id=AJPIAS000070000012001259000001&idtype=cvips [Accessed June 16, 2009].
13. USDE. 2003. U.S. Department of Education, Identifying and Implementing Educational Practices Supported by Rigorous Evidence: A User Friendly Guide. Institute of Education Sciences, National Center for Education

Evaluation and Regional Assistance. The entire guide is online at <http://www.ed.gov/rschstat/research/pubs/rigorousevid/index.html> / "PDF (140KB)".

14. Shadish, W.R., T.D. Cook, & D.T. Campbell. 2002. Experimental and Quasi-Experimental Designs for Generalized Causal Inference. Houghton Mifflin - information at <http://tinyurl.com/y3e7vw>.
15. Colt HG, Davoudi M, Murgu SD, Zamanian Rohani N. Colt HG, Davoudi M, Murgu S, and Rohani NZ. Measuring learning gain during a one-day introductory bronchoscopy course. Surgical Endoscopy 2010;25:207-216.
16. Colt HG, Davoudi M, Quadrelli S, Rohani N. Competency-based metrics to measure short-term knowledge and skill acquisition during a two-day thoracoscopy program. Respiration 2010;80(6):553-559.

Introduction to Flexible Bronchoscopy

One day program with didactic lectures, interactive sessions, and hands-on workshops. Example of program objectives and methods.

Program Objectives

At the end of this one-day program that includes didactic, interactive, and hands-on training sessions, the program participant will have:

- Increased factual knowledge of flexible bronchoscopy as it pertains to:
    - Patient safety, prevention and response to complications
    - Special populations
    - Airway anatomy, brushing, biopsy, TBLB, and conventional TBNA
    - Evaluation of central airway disorders
- Enhanced medical decision-making ability
- Improved technical skill performing bronchoscopy inspection, brushing, biopsy conventional TBNA, and emergency bronchoscopically-guided endotracheal intubation.

Methods used to accomplish program objectives

- Didactic lectures (8 sessions) might also be interactive when flipped classroom is used.
- Interactive sessions (3 sessions)
- Patient-centered problem-based learning exercises (1 session)
- Hands-on technical skill training using inanimate airway models and computer-based simulation, (4 sessions).
- Instructor-led small group interactive exercises pertaining to diagnostic bronchoscopic strategies, informed consent and patient safety (at least 1 session).
- Assessment of technical skill performing bronchoscopic inspection using validated bronchoscopy assessment tools (BSAT and BSTAT) if time allows.
- Post course written knowledge assessment with general review of correct answers.

Example of Course Schedule (Southern California, with participation of 7 different training institutions)

One day Introductory Bronchoscopy Course for First Year Pulmonary and Critical care Medicine Trainees

7:30-8:15 am	Registration, pre-course technical skill assessments
8:15-8:30	Welcome, introduction, and learning objectives
8:30-9:00	Pretest and survey of practice experience
9:00-9:20	Patient safety: Pre-bronchoscopy evaluation
9:20-9:40	Patient safety: Bronchoscopy in special populations
9:40-10:15	Preventing and managing airway complications
10:15-10:30	BREAK
10:30-10:45	Anatomic relationships
10:45-11:15	Bronchoscopic airway inspection
11:15-11:45	Evaluation of central airway obstruction
11:45-12:00	Basic diagnostic procedures (lavage, brushings, and biopsy)
12:00-12:30	Transbronchial lung biopsy
12:30-1:00	Practical approach to transbronchial needle aspiration
1:00-2:00	LUNCH
Afternoon hands-on training 2:00-4:30 pm	Hands-on training: 5 stations - 30 minutes per station (1) Airway anatomy and bronchoscopy step by step (2) Endobronchial brushings, and endobronchial biopsy (3) Transbronchial needle aspiration (4) Emergency bronchoscopic intubation (5) Diagnostic strategies: interactive small group session
4:30-4:45	Post course technical skills learning assessment
4:45-5:15	Post course cognitive learning assessment
5:15-5:30	Interactive session: True-False exercices
5:30-6:00 pm	Wrap up; certificate of course completion

Introduction to Flexible Bronchoscopy: Hands-On Workstations

Workstation 1: Airway Anatomy & Bronchoscopy Step by Step©

Learning Objectives:

1. To be able to enter the airway from the larynx atraumatically and navigate down the trachea maintaining the bronchoscope in the midline.
2. To learn to practice the initial "right-left" maneuver.
3. To become familiar with right-sided exercises.
4. To become familiar with left-sided exercises.
5. To be able to identify bronchial segmental anatomy, and to understand the order of segmental airway examination.

Description:

The instructor will first demonstrate step by step principles and techniques of airway examination. Learners will then use simulation to study bronchial anatomy, and focus on principles that include keeping the scope in the midline, avoiding wall trauma (red out), identifying and entering bronchial segments appropriately, and performing certain left and right sided exercises. Following the performance principles of Decision-Intention-Control, and Economy of movement, learners will develop muscle memory and elegance through guided repetition and focused practice.

Workstation 2: Endobronchial Brushing & Endobronchial Biopsy

Learning Objectives:

1. To be able to brush a simulation of a mucosal lesion using proper communication skills and technique while maintaining the bronchoscope in the midline and without causing airway trauma.
2. To be able to biopsy a simulation of a mucosal lesion using proper communication skills and technique while maintaining the bronchoscope in the midline and without causing airway trauma.

Description:

The instructor will guide the learner as the learner brushes and biopsies an airway abnormality. Another learner may serve as the bronchoscopy assistant, so that the "bronchoscopist" may practice and learn proper communication skills such as "brush out, brush in, open forceps, close forceps" while maintaining proper bronchoscopic technique.

Workstation 3: Transbronchial Needle Aspiration

Learning Objectives:

1. To be able to demonstrate three different techniques of needle insertion: hub against wall, piggy-back, and jab technique.
2. To be able to demonstrate three ways to protect the bronchoscope during needle aspiration: Straightening the scope during needle insertion and removal, complete visualization of the needle during retraction from the airway wall, pulling the needle completely into the sheath before removal through the bronchoscope.

Description:

The instructor will first demonstrate videobronchoscopy and each of the three techniques of TBNA with the help of a bronchoscopy assistant. TBNA will be performed through the carina into subcarinal adenopathy of the specially lo-fidelity airway model. The instructor will also describe different ways with which to assure patient and operator safely, and ways in which the flexible bronchoscope is protected. Each team member will then demonstrate needle insertion techniques, while another team member serves as the bronchoscopy assistant, making certain that patient, operator, and equipment safety are assured.

Workstation 4: Difficult Airway: Emergency Bronchoscopic Intubation

Learning Objectives:

1. The learner should be able to manage a normal, emergency airway, using mask ventilation, laryngoscopic intubation, and fiberoptic intubation.
2. The learner should be able to intubate a patient with a difficult airway (limited jaw range of motion, swollen tongue) using the flexible bronchoscope

Description:

Intubation in the patient with a difficult airway is a life-saving procedure. Family members, nursing teams, physicians, and respiratory therapists are often watching or assisting at the bedside. It is a time for the bronchoscopist to take control of the situation while using the airway team wisely in order to maintain an effective, calm and trusting environment.

Workstation 5: Diagnostic Strategies: Interactive Small Group Session

Learning Objectives:

1. The learner should be able to proceed through the 4-Box Patient-centered practical approach method, knowing the significance of each box.
2. The learner should be able to analyze a bronchoscopic case by walking a colleague through the process of initial patient evaluation, assessment of procedural strategies, discussion of procedural techniques and results, and devising long-term management plans.

Description:

In this interactive session, the instructor opens the floor to the learners, and together they walk through a complicated case using the 4-Box Practical Approach model, working their way through initial patient evaluation, assessment of procedural strategies (including indications and contraindications, expected results, and risk-benefit analysis), discussion of procedural techniques and results (including choosing among technical options and instruments, knowing the anatomic risks, results, and possible complications and how to deal with each), and devising long-term management plans (including assessment of the results, plan for follow-up diagnostic and therapeutic options, along with quality improvement for the procedural team).

References

1. Davoudi M, Colt HG. Bronchoscopy simulation: a brief review. Adv Health Sci Educ 2009;14:287-296.
2. Goldberg R, Colt HG, Davoudi M, Cherisson L. Realistic and affordable lo-fidelity model for learning transbronchial needle aspiration. Surg Endosc 2009;23(9):2047-52.
3. Davoudi M, Wahidi MM, Rohani NZ, Colt HG. Comparative effectiveness of low and high-fidelity bronchoscopy simulation for training in conventional transbronchial needle aspiration and user preferences. Respiration 2010;80:327-334.
4. Ost D, DeRosiers A, Britt EJ, et al. Assessment of a bronchoscopy simulator. Am J Respir Crit Care Med 2001;164(12):2248-55.
5. Crawford SW and Colt HG. Virtual reality and written assessments are of potential value to determine knowledge and skill in flexible bronchoscopy. Respiration 2004; 71:269 – 275.
6. Colt HG, Crawford, SW., Galbraith O. Virtual reality bronchoscopy simulation: A revolution in procedural training. Chest 2001; 120(4):1333–1339.
7. Colt HG, Davoudi M, Murgu S, and Rohani NZ. Measuring learning gain during a one-day introductory bronchoscopy course. Surg Endoscopy 2010;25:207-216.
8. Wahidi MM, Silvestri GA, Coakley RD, Ferguson JS, Shepherd RW, Moses L, Conforti J, Que L, Anstrom KJ, McGuire F, Colt H, Downie GH. A prospective multi-center study of competency metrics and educational interventions in the learning of bronchoscopy among starting pulmonary fellows. Chest 2010;137(5):1040-1049.

Introduction to Flexible Bronchoscopy
20 Question Post-test

Please choose only ONE answer for each of the following questions.

1. Which of the following statements about bronchoalveolar lavage (BAL) is <u>true</u>:
   a. BAL-induced hypoxemia is a sign of poor operator technique
   b. BAL fluid return is greater in smokers than in nonsmokers.
   c. It is standard of care to exclude the first aliquot containing mostly bronchial cells
   d. RML, lingula and the lower lobes are preferred sites due to optimal fluid return
   e. BAL may provide diagnosis in up to 25 percent of patients with peripheral endoscopically non-visible lesions.

2. Which of the following statements about endobronchial biopsy is <u>true</u>:
   a. Suspicion of sarcoidosis, despite normal mucosa, is an accepted indication
   b. The jaws of the biopsy forceps must be at least 2 cm. from the distal end of the bronchoscope at the time of biopsy
   c. Cup forceps should always be used rather than alligator forceps.
   d. Pre-procedure measurements of PT, PTT, and platelet count are necessary
   e. Biopsy should be avoided in patients on aspirin

3. Which of the following statements about endobronchial brushing is <u>true</u>:
   a. The use of fluoroscopy for endobronchial brushing is strongly recommended
   b. Yield for peripheral malignant lesions has consistently been reported over 50%
   c. Yield for central lesions is frequently greater than 50%
   d. Pneumothorax or bleeding occur in 1-4 % of cases.
   e. If brushing and BAL are combined for diagnosis of malignancy, BAL must always be performed first to diminish Red Blood Cell contamination of specimen

4. Procedure-related morbidity and mortality occur most frequently after which procedure:

a. Transbronchial biopsy
b. Endobronchial biopsy
c. Endobronchial brushing
d. Transbronchial needle aspiration
e. Endobronchial needle aspiration

5. Which statement is true regarding bronchospasm and laryngospasm:

a. Acute bronchospasm is a contraindication to bronchoscopy
b. For laryngospasm, racemic epinephrine should be given every 3 minutes until laryngospasm has resolved
c. Patients with COPD should receive bronchodilators before flexible bronchoscopy.
d. The administration of topical anesthesia always diminishes the risk of laryngospasm
e. Premedication of asthmatic patients with bronchodilator is not recommended

6. Which of the following statements about bronchoscopy-related pneumothorax is true:

a. It is only seen after transbronchial biopsy
b. It is seen more commonly when biopsying central lesions
c. The usual initial presentation is subcutaneous emphysema
d. Observation rather than small bore chest tube insertion is warranted if small and asymptomatic
e. Chest radiographs should be obtained routinely after bronchoscopy with transbronchial biopsy

7. Which statement is false about measures to prevent bleeding after transbronchial biopsies in a high risk patient:

a. Stop oral anti-coagulation at least 3 days prior to bronchoscopy
b. Hold Plavix (clopidogrel) 5-7 days prior to bronchoscopy
c. In thrombocytopenia, transfuse up to > 15,000 /mm3
d. Check PT/PTT/Platelet count in patients with prior history of bleeding or coagulopathy
e. Discuss the increased risk with the patient during the informed consent process

8. You perform a transbronchial lung biopsy, and see blood coming out of the biopsied segment. The first thing you do is:

a. Turn patient to the lateral decubitus position to protect the contralateral lung
b. Immediate unilateral intubation over the bronchoscope
c. Large bore suctioning of the oropharynx
d. Use washes of cold saline or saline with epinephrine
e. Directly tamponade the bleeding airway using the wedged bronchoscope

9. In which of the following should you avoid performing diagnostic bronchoscopy with BAL:

a. Elevated intracranial pressure
b. Acute coronary syndrome
c. Impending respiratory failure
d. Severe pulmonary hypertension
e. Severe COPD

10. Which action is <u>not recommended</u> to treat hypoxemia in a patient during bronchoscopy-related bleeding:

a. Administration of high flow oxygen through mask
b. Oropharyngeal suctioning
c. Improving airflow by removal of clots from the bleeding segmental airway
d. Lateral decubitus positioning with bleeding side down
e. Frequent suctioning of blood from "the good side"

11. Patients with asthma should receive pre-procedure bronchodilators:

a. Only if they are wheezing on examination
b. Only if you are going to perform bronchoscopic biopsies
c. Only if they are known to have an FEV1 less than 40 % predicted
d. Routinely, even for inspection bronchoscopy
e. Only if they are on inhaled or oral corticosteroids

12. Which of the following <u>does not</u> preclude transbronchial biopsy:

a. ASA 325 mg q day
b. Warfarin 5 mg po q day
c. Enoxeparin sq 1 mg/kg bid
d. Clopidogrel 75 mg po q day
e. Heparin intravenous bolus for suspected pulmonary embolism three hours earlier

13. TBNA of the right lower paratracheal lymph node station [station 4R] is performed

a. Two centimeters above the carina along the antero-lateral wall of the trachea
b. Two centimeters above the carina along the postero-lateral wall of the trachea
c. At the level of the carina along the lateral wall of the trachea
d. At the level of the carina along the posterolateral wall of the trachea
e. At the level of the carina along the anterolateral wall of the trachea

14. According to the American Thoracic Society guidelines, which of the following is an absolute contraindication to flexible bronchoscopy:

a. Recent myocardial infarction
b. Refractory hypercarbia with altered mental status
c. Severe refractory hypoxemia during bronchoscopy
d. Status asthmaticus during bronchoscopy
e. Acute superior vena cava obstruction

15. Which of the following is not an expected BAL-related adverse event?

a. Hypoxemia
b. Fever
c. Increased infiltrates on chest radiograph
d. Worsening respiratory insufficiency
e. Hemoptysis

16. Which of the statements regarding saber sheath trachea is true:

a. It is seen in up to twenty percent of asthmatics
b. It is seen in up to one third of elderly patients
c. It is seen in up to five percent of COPD patients, with no clinical significance
d. It is common in patients with long-standing Wegener's Granulomatosis
e. It is more common in Asians, compared to Caucasians or Blacks.

17. Two hours after performing BAL and transbronchial lung biopsies from the right lower lobe in a patient with focal lung infiltrates, your patient complains of right pleuritic chest discomfort. You should:

a. Examine the patient and if normal, discharge home with instructions for follow-up by telephone later that day.
b. Examine the patient and if abnormal, consider insertion of a small bore chest tube
c. Examine the patient and obtain an expiratory chest radiograph
d. Examine the patient and obtain an expiratory chest radiograph if the exam is abnormal
e. Examine the patient, and insert a large bore chest tube if abnormal

18. Massive bleeding occurs immediately after transbronchial lung biopsy from the lateral basal segment of the left lower lobe. You should immediately:

a. Withdraw the bronchoscope to the carina to protect the contralateral airway
b. Wedge the bronchoscope into the bleeding segment and suction continuously
c. Turn the patient onto the right lateral decubitus position
d. Turn the patient onto the left lateral decubitus position
e. Administer additional sedation to relax the patient and control the cough reflex induced by blood.

19. Transbronchial lung biopsy has the lowest yield for the diagnosis of which of the following:

a. Usual interstitial pneumonia (UIP)
b. Sarcoidosis
c. Acute eosinophilic pneumonia
d. Lymphangitic carcinomatosis
e. Goodpasture's syndrome

20. The use of fluoroscopy during bronchoscopy is least likely to achieve which of the following:

a. To diminish the risk of bleeding with transbronchial lung biopsy
b. To increase the yield of transbronchial biopsy of a localized lesion
c. To diminish the risk of pneumothorax in transbronchial lung biopsy
d. To increase the yield of brushing in a solitary pulmonary nodule
e. To increase the yield of retrieval of a 5 mm. foreign body

Introduction to Flexible Bronchoscopy

Answers

Correct responses for twenty question post-test

1. E	2. A	3. C	4. A	5. A	6. D	7. C	8. E	9. C	10. C
11. D	12. A	13. A	14. C	15. E	16. C	17. C	18. D	19. A	20. A

Introduction to Flexible Bronchoscopy

Course Evaluation Form

A. Please indicate your position: (Circle) Trainee Practitioner Full-time Faculty

B. How well did this activity meet the following learning objectives? (Circle one)

(Scale for B: 1=not at all, 2=slightly, 3=moderately, 4=mostly, 5=completely)

Course Objectives					
Increased my factual knowledge of flexible bronchoscopy particularly as it pertains to patient safety (such as indications, prevention and response to complications)	1	2	3	4	5
Increased my knowledge of flexible bronchoscopy particularly as it pertains to special populations	1	2	3	4	5
Increased my knowledge of bronchoscopic procedures: biopsy, lavage, brushing, transbronchial biopsy and conventional transbronchial needle aspiration	1	2	3	4	5
Increased my decision-making ability using patient-centered case scenarios	1	2	3	4	5
Improved my understanding and memory of bronchial anatomy	1	2	3	4	5
Improved my technical skill regarding performance of bronchoscopic airway inspection	1	2	3	4	5
Improved my technical skill regarding performance of bronchoscopic brushing and/or biopsy	1	2	3	4	5
Improved my technical skill regarding conventional transbronchial needle aspiration	1	2	3	4	5
Improved my technical skill regarding emergency bronchoscopic endotracheal intubation	1	2	3	4	5

C. **Please rate each of the following presentations based on content, literature review, and objectivity Also, please rate each of the presenters based on communication skills, ability to keep your attention, and clarity**

(Scale for C: 1=Needs improvement, 2=below average, 3=average, 4=above average, 5=outstanding)

Presentations	Presenter	Communication Skills	Content, Objectivity & Scientific Rigor
Patient Safety: Prebronchoscopy Evaluation	xx	1 2 3 4 5	1 2 3 4 5
Patient Safety: Bronchoscopy in Special Populations	xx	1 2 3 4 5	1 2 3 4 5
Preventing and Managing Airway Complications	xx	1 2 3 4 5	1 2 3 4 5
Bronchoscopic Airway Inspection	xx	1 2 3 4 5	1 2 3 4 5
Anatomic Relationships	xx	1 2 3 4 5	1 2 3 4 5
Evaluation of Central Airway Obstruction	xx	1 2 3 4 5	1 2 3 4 5
Bronchoscopic Washing, Brushing & Biopsy	xx	1 2 3 4 5	1 2 3 4 5
Transbronchial Lung Biopsy	xx	1 2 3 4 5	1 2 3 4 5
Transbronchial Needle Aspiration	xx	1 2 3 4 5	1 2 3 4 5

D. **Workshops: Please rate each of the following Hands-on workshops based on quality of training**

(Scale for D: 1=Needs improvement, 2=below average, 3=average, 4=above average, 5=outstanding)

Workshop	Instructor	Mentor Skills	Training Methods and Models used
Airway Anatomy and Bronchoscopy Step by Step	xx	1 2 3 4 5	1 2 3 4 5
Endobronchial Brushings and Biopsies	xx	1 2 3 4 5	1 2 3 4 5
Conventional Transbronchial needle Aspiration	xx	1 2 3 4 5	1 2 3 4 5
Emergency Bronchoscopic Intubation	xx	1 2 3 4 5	1 2 3 4 5
Bronchoscopic strategies/patient-centered approach	xx	1 2 3 4 5	1 2 3 4 5

E. **Logistics and Facilities: Please rate each of the following based on your preferences**

(Scale for E: 1 =Inadequate, 2=below average, 3=average, 4=above average, 5=outstanding)

Logistical Items					
Facilities: Lecture Room	1	2	3	4	5
Facilities: Workshop Rooms	1	2	3	4	5
Food Service	1	2	3	4	5

F. **Length of activity: _______ Too short _______ Satisfactory _______ Too long**

G. **Was this seminar valuable? _______ Yes _______No**

H. **What might we do to make this seminar better?**

____

____

____

____

____

Thank you for participating in this seminar and for completing this evaluation. We appreciate your input and hope you found the lectures, workshops and time we spent together helpful.

The Bronchoscopy International Team and Guest Faculty

SECTION 2

Reading Assignments

- *The Essential Flexible Bronchoscopist©* modules 1-6
- *Moderate Sedation* module
- *Fluoroscopy* module

USER INSTRUCTIONS

For modules 1-6 of the Essential Flexible Bronchoscopist© with post-tests

The web-based, hardcopy and electronic version Essential Bronchoscopist™ series contains books pertaining to the art, science and practice of bronchoscopy. The first in the series is The Essential Flexible Bronchoscopist©. This is a laddered curriculum of theoretic bronchoscopic knowledge that can be accessed free of charge in 14 languages including English, French, Spanish, Portuguese, Turkish, Vietnamese, Japanese, Korean, and Chinese. As mentioned previously, this text is also available in electronic and printed form. It has been officially endorsed as a complementary educational tool by several national and international bronchology and pulmonary organizations (including for example those from Argentina, Singapore, Hungary, Peru, Italy, Indonesia, Belgium, Malaysia, Spain, France, Brazil, Korea, and Japan, as well as by the American Association for Bronchology, The South American Association for Bronchoesophagology, and the World Association for Bronchology and Interventional Pulmonology). The essential-bronchoscopy.com website is HONcode certified (Health on the Net), and can also be accessed through the Bronchoscopy International website at www.bronchoscopy.org.

The Essential Flexible Bronchoscopist© deconstructs procedures into three major elements: strategy and planning, technical skills, and outcomes assessment (quality control and ability to respond to complications). In order to identify the elements crucial to medical reasoning when entertaining a bronchoscopy consultation, these elements are further deconstructed into four categories using a four-box practical approach to procedural decision making: patient evaluation, procedural strategies, techniques, and outcomes described in one of the six elements of the Essential Bronchoscopist™ curriculum; the patient-centered practical approach to procedural decision making.

This curriculum is used as a foundation for a more uniform curricula delivered by experienced volunteer bronchoscopy educators who have participated in specially designed faculty development programs (train the trainers) established by Bronchoscopy International, in order to provide regional seminars in countries around the world.

The Essential Flexible Bronchoscopist© is comprised of six modules, each with a module-specific competency-based learning objective, totaling 186 multiple-choice question-answer sets. Each question-answer set contains information pertaining to the major topics represented in traditional textbooks of bronchoscopy (anatomy and airway abnormalities, patient preparation, indications, contraindications and complications, techniques and solutions to technical problems, lung cancer and infections, bronchoalveolar lavage, lung biopsy techniques, therapeutic and interventional bronchoscopy, anesthesia and medications, equipment and its maintenance, as well as history and education).

The aim of The Essential Bronchoscopist© series is not to replace but to complement the conventional apprenticeship model of training in bronchoscopy by emphasizing important facets of knowledge and skill required for competency, and by encouraging trainees to discuss these with their preceptors and colleagues[i]. Elements addressed in The Essential Flexible Bronchoscopist© are intentionally written so that contrary opinions might occasionally be provided by instructors. In this fashion, dialogue is promoted, but access to a certain amount of "essential" material is guaranteed. In one study, conducted in Argentina and the USA, select material from the question-answer sets of The Essential Flexible Bronchoscopist©, were used to create a validated test of bronchoscopic knowledge. Questions from The Essential Flexible Bronchoscopist© have also been used in other studies pertaining to bronchoscopy education and low-stakes examinations.

In order to document that a learner has been exposed to material contained in The Essential Flexible Bronchoscopist©, a passing score on each of the post-tests is warranted. If completed on-line, learners with unsatisfactory grades can take the test three times before they automatically are allowed to proceed to the next module. All learners should document a passing score as proof that they have completed the module. A score of 70 and above (7 correct responses) allows the learner to move on to the next module using the online version. After three attempts, the next module can be accessed regardless of one's score. A hardcopy print-out of one's passing scores can be placed in the learner's file so that program directors can check off the module as completed on the Introduction to Flexible Bronchoscopy Program Completion Checklist. A copy of the post-test questions is included in this training manual, as well as answers for each module's post-test. Learners are encouraged to read the module's question and answer sets prior to taking the module's post test. An honor system is assumed in regards to each learner's refraining from viewing post-test answer sheets prior to reading the module and taking the post-test.

Selected References

1. Colt HG, Davoudi M, Quadrelli S. Pilot study of web-based bronchoscopy education using the Essential Bronchoscopist in developing countries (Mauritania and Mozambique). Respiration 2007;74:358-359.
2. Colt HG, Ngoc van Tran, Quadrelli S, than Pham van. Creation of an interventional technical plateau at Cho ray Hospital, Vietnam. J Bronchol 2007;14:289-292.
3. Davoudi M, Quadrelli S, Osann K, and Colt HG. A competency-based test of bronchoscopic knowledge using the Essential Bronchoscopist: an initial concept study. Respirology, 2008;13:736-743.
4. Quadrelli S, Galíndez F, Davoudi M Colt HG,. Reliability of a 25 item *low stakes* multiple choice assessment of bronchoscopic knowledge. Chest 2009;135:315-321.
5. Wahidi MM, Silvestri GA, Coakley RD, Ferguson JS, Shepherd RW, Moses L, Conforti J, Que L, Anstrom KJ, McGuire F, Colt H, Downie GH. A prospective multi-center study of competency metrics and educational interventions in the learning of bronchoscopy among starting pulmonary fellows. Chest 2010;137(5):1040-1049.

[i] Other elements of this series include The Essential EBUS Bronchoscopist, The Essential cTBNA Bronchoscopist, and The Essential Intensivist Bronchoscopist.

USER INSTRUCTIONS

Moderate Sedation and Fluoroscopy Modules

The purpose of these readings is to provide learners with exposure to major principles pertaining to the use of moderate sedation and fluoroscopy during bronchoscopy. While many institutions have regulations and bronchoscopy-related protocols, many are without a formal program of education in these areas.

The inappropriate use of medications and fluoroscopy can severely affect patient safety. This is why we have designed a series of checklists to help enhance patient safety and to document the acquisition of knowledge in these areas during the course of training.

We recommend at least ONE formal session during which a didactic lecture on each of these two subjects is provided after learners have reviewed the synopsis and other reading material. Checklists can be reviewed at separate individual or group sessions, or during the course of day-to-day procedural training.

Moderate Sedation: Synopsis

The purpose of this synopsis is to provide the reader with a brief overview of moderate sedation as it might apply to flexible bronchoscopy. It is assumed that institutions and practitioners have different biases and regulations. Herein a short summary is provided so that beginner bronchoscopists might acquire at least some of the elements necessary for a safe procedure. Readers are encouraged to follow guidelines and protocols established in their own institutions.

Definitions

- Moderate sedation may be produced by the use of intravenous, oral, transmucosal or intramuscular narcotics, sedatives or anxiolytic medications
- Moderate sedation is a medically controlled state of depressed consciousness that allows protective reflexes to be maintained, while retaining the patient's ability to maintain a patent airway independently and continuously. This implies that the patient is mildly drowsy but arouses to voice easily. This is to be distinguished from
- Deep sedation, where the patient is arousable only by vigorous stimulation and may lose the ability to maintain airway patency and protection.

ASA Classification

- ASA 1: normal and healthy patient
- ASA 2: Mild controlled systemic disease and no functional limitation
- ASA 3: Moderate to severe systemic disease that limits activity.
- ASA 4: severe systemic disease that is a constant threat to life or is functionally incapacitating.
- ASA 5: Moribund and not expected to survive without surgery

Equipment

- Informed consent for sedation should be obtained in addition to consent for the procedure.
- Oximetry
- Ability to monitor the patient for vital signs, airway patency, degree of wakefulness.

- Electrocardiogram
- Intravenous access
- Rescue equipment for any patient moving into deep sedation, including crash cart and defibrillator
- Appropriate size endotracheal tubes and ability to ventilate patient (including self-inflating Ambu-bag and mask system) should be available.
- Reversal agents for narcotics and benzodiazepines
- Charting should include baseline ventilatory, hemodynamic, neurologic status, time of administration of medication, dose administered, type of medication used, physical examination, informed consent, allergies, nothing to eat 8 hours prior to the procedure (except for clear liquids and medications, up to four hours prior to procedure).
- Ability to monitor patient status at least every 15 minutes during the procedure and for a minimum of thirty (30) minutes after the procedure and/or until patient returns to baseline status, including pulse oximetry equal or greater than 92% on room air, or assured with supplemental oxygen if patient on oxygen.
- Following administration of reversal agents such as naloxone, patient should not be discharged for a minimum of one (1) hour, and flumazenil two (2) hours.

Potential contraindications

- Uncooperative patients
- Mentally ill patients
- Severe cardiac, pulmonary, hepatic, renal or central nervous disease
- Pregnancy
- Morbid obesity
- Alcohol or drug abuse
- History of sleep apnea

High risk patients

- Previous problems with anesthesia or sedation
- Previous surgery or radiation or injury to neck or face
- Stridor, snoring, or sleep apnea
- Dysmorphic facial features
- Advanced rheumatoid arthritis
- Significant obesity, protruding teeth
- Small mouth opening (<3cm in adults), macroglossia, non-visible uvula, tonsillar hypertrophy, short neck, limited neck extension, decreased hyoid-mental distance (<3cm in adult).

Response to complications

- Ability to rotate patient onto lateral decubitus position in case of vomiting.
- Ability to insert a nasal trumpet
- Ability to perform chin lift/neck extension in case of obstructed airway
- Oral suction should always be available
- Ability to establish a safe and patent airway, and provide hemodynamic and circulatory support in case of compromise.

Specific medications

- *Midazolam* (Versed) is currently the most widely used agent for moderate sedation and anxiolysis. It is a water-soluble benzodiazepine with rapid onset of action. It is four times more potent on a mg per mg basis than
    - o When administered intravenously, sedation and anxiolysis usually occurs within 2 minutes. Complete recovery of motor performance and consciousness occurs within one hour in most individuals.
    - o Combining Midazolam and opioides increases the incidence of apnea. Large doses can produce prolonged drowsiness and cardio-respiratory arrest. Central nervous system dysfunction, including confusion and seizures can be seen in patients with brain metastases and paraneoplastic syndromes.
    - o Ventilation is depressed by 0.15 mg/kg, especially in patients with COPD. The peak effect of respiratory depression occurs at three minutes following injection and remains for approximately 15 minutes. It can be most pronounced in geriatric and COPD patients.
- *Fentanyl* is a synthetic opiate analog that is structurally different from morphine or meperidine. It is 100 times more potent than morphine. The usual adult dose is 50-100 micrograms. Given intravenously, its onset of action and maximum respiratory depression effect occurs about 5-10 minutes after administration, and lasts 30-60 minutes.
    - o Given intramuscularly, the onset of action is within 7-15 minutes with duration of action lasting up to two hours.
    - o Fentanyl should never be used in patients receiving MAO inhibitors because of increased risk of respiratory depression and coma.
- *Combination drugs.* Sedative responses are increased in patients who have received opioides or other benzodiazepines. Level of sedation and risk for respiratory depression are increased in the elderly and in patients with pre-existing respiratory dysfunction.
- *Reversal agents*:
    - o Naloxone is a pure opiate antagonist that reverses all effects and side effects of opiates.). The initial dose is 0.1-0.2 mg IV, SQ, IM or via endotracheal tube and can be repeated every 2 minutes. The onset of action is about 30 seconds. Actually, no more than 0.4 mg should be administered because this might lead to increased activity of the sympathetic nervous system

from acute termination of analgesia. Consequently, patients may develop hypertension, dysrhythmias, and pulmonary edema.

- Flumazenil is a benzodiazepine antagonist that should be administered (0.2 mg IV over 15 seconds, then repeated every minute up to a maximum of 1 mg). Low doses of Flumazenil will reliably reverse sedation within 2 minutes, but higher doses are needed to reverse benzodiazepine-related anxiolysis. Duration of action is about 60 minutes. Side effects include nausea, vomiting, tremors, seizures, tears and dizziness. Contrary to naloxone, it does not cause hemodynamic instability.

Dosing guidelines

- *Midazolam* single dose 1 mg IV, onset of action 1-2.5 minutes, total dose 5 mg
- *Lorazapam* single dose 2 mg IV, onset of action 20-30 minutes, total dose 4 mg
- *Morphine* single dose 2-4 mg IV, onset of action 1-5 minutes, total dose 10 mg
- *Fentanyl* single dose 50 mcg IV, onset of action 1-5 min, total dose 100 mcg

Fluoroscopy: Synopsis

The purpose of this synopsis is to provide the reader with a brief overview of fluoroscopy as it might apply to flexible bronchoscopy. It is assumed that institutions and practitioners have different biases and regulations. Herein a short summary is provided so that beginner bronchoscopists might acquire at least some of the elements necessary for a safe procedure. Readers are encouraged to follow guidelines and protocols established in their own institutions. Students are urged to read the Syllabus on Fluoroscopy and Radiation Protection created by the California Department of Health Services, which is downloadable from http://www.cdph.ca.gov/pubsforms/Guidelines/Documents/RHB-FluoroSyllabus.pdf

Definitions and consequences

- Refraction is the bending of light rays as they pass from a medium of one density to a medium of a different density. Brightness improves visual acuity
  - If the fluoroscopic image is not bright enough to be of good quality, it cannot be improved by prolonged observation.
- Visual acuity is the ability of the eye to recognized differences between two sources of light stimulus, and thus to perceive fine detail.
  - Night vision is best when the eye scans a scene (moving the fluoroscopic image).
- The eye retains any image it receives for a fraction of a second after the image is removed.
  - Frame rates of 24 frames per second (still frames as for television), will thus appear continuous, as in a movie).
- Fluoroscopy images are electromagnetic radiation waves traveling at the speed of light (186,000 miles/second). Photons have energy that is directly proportional to the frequency or inversely proportional to the wavelength of the radiation.
  - Increasing voltage increases energy and shortens the wavelength, making a more energetic and penetrating beam. The intensity of the radiation beam is influenced by current (milliAmperes mA).

- Radiation, like all energy, can be primary, scattered, or remnant. Interactions with tissues continue until all energies are spent.
  - Primary is the radiation emitted directly towards the patient, scattered is what happens when the energy collides with matter (the patient), remnant is the energy that pass through the patient and strikes the image detector.
- Scatter increases if tissue density or thickness increases, or when voltage and milliAmperage increase.
  - Compton scatter results from colliding electrons that lose their energy, as photons are scattered in all directions at low energies. Usually this is associated with increased voltage, and will diminish the quality of the fluoroscopic image. This causes quantum mottle (a grainy appearance in the image)
- Resolution, Distortion, and Lag time
  - Definitions provided below. Move fluoroscope slowly while scanning. Keep image centered, and use highest lines/mm monitor (screen) possible.

Reducing patient exposure

- Collimate (focus) the radiation beam to the target of interest
- Use last image hold technique of fluoroscopy rather than continuous applications
- Keep patient to image intensifier (image to detector) distance as short as possible. Moving image intensifier away from the patient increases patient radiation dose.
- Use highest voltage and lowest milliAmperage as possible
- Use largest image intensifier mode (with non magnification) if possible
- Target to tabletop distance never less than 12 inches (30 cm), and should be at least 18 inches (45 cm) because patient dose decreases with increasing distance
- Use low absorption tabletops (made of aluminum, Bakelite, or carbon fiber) that do not attenuate the radiation beam.
- Use "dead-man" exposure switch (pedal) that terminates the radiation exposure when the foot is removed from the pedal. Do not provide continuous exposure.
- Doubling exposure time doubles radiation dose to both operator and patient.
- Do not use magnification mode unless absolutely necessary.

Improving visibility

- Adjust brightness and contrast settings on the screen
- Darken the procedure room lighting
- Avoid changing settings such as milliAmperage or voltage. It is better to adjust room lighting and screen properties.
- Changing the brightness setting on the screen will not improve quality of original image.

- Changing the contrast mode on the screen should be set so that bright objects of interest do not completely saturate (white out). It may be necessary to modify brightness after changing contrast modes.

Patient and operator shielding and monitoring

- Gonad shields, Thyroid shields
- Lead curtains, Body aprons
- Personal radiation film badges should be worn at collar height above the protective apron or on top of the protective apron itself.
- Badges should be checked periodically to record exposure and measure accumulated exposure over a specified period of time

Special precautions for pregnant patient and health care providers

- There is always a potential for adverse biological effects after exposure to radiation.
- Examinations should not be postponed if deemed clinically necessary, but appropriate shielding precautions should be followed.
- There is no “safe” period” for the real or potential embryo/fetus or future fertilized ovum
- Therapeutic abortion is never justified because of radiation dose to embryo/fetus during a diagnostic fluoroscopic examination
- Effects are proportional to absorbed radiation dose
- The first three months of pregnancy are when the embryo-fetus is most sensitive to radiation.
- Pregnant or potentially pregnant health care providers should not assist in fluoroscopic procedures.

Resolution, Distortion, Scattered radiation, and Lag

- Limited by screen capabilities (525 to 1000 lines/mm)
- Defined as the ability of the imaging system to differentiate small objects as separate images when they are close together.
- Distortion effects size and shape, and can be greatest at the periphery of the image.
- Lag time, and thus blurring of the image as the fluoroscope is moved, occurs because it takes a certain amount of time for the image to build on the screen.
- Scattered radiation is increased in case of high voltage, large field size and thick body parts (obesity.
- The fluoroscopist and assistants should stand as far away from the patient as possible.
- The dose of radiation received from scattered radiation by the fluoroscopist and assistants is directly proportional to the patient radiation dose.
- Preferably a 0.5 mm protective apron should be worn (transmitted exposure reduction is thus 99.9 percent, as compared to 97% reduction for a 0.25 mm apron). Aprons cover only 80% of active bone marrow of the body.

Basic operational procedures

- Use short looks rather than continuous observation. Because the recognition time of the human eye is 0.2 seconds, a short look will accomplish the same as continuous observation.
- Use a resettable timer that will alarm when a maximum of 5 minutes exposure time is reached.
- Use best contrast (lowest milliAmperage) and highest peak voltage possible.
- Keep target area small and focused, but without magnification mode.
- Maintain radiation dose as low as possible (should be less than 5 rads per minute)
- Use last frame hold strategy to keep an image on screen without additional radiation exposure.
- Place image intensifier as close to the patient as possible.
- Prevent patient motion by giving clear instructions.
- Reduce extraneous light in procedure room.
- Use gonad shields and protective aprons of at least 0.25 mm lead equivalent.
- Use audible indicator (beeper alert) when fluoroscopy is on.
- Use personal radiation dose monitoring devices (radiation badge) according to institutional guidelines.

SECTION 3

Bronchoscopy Step-by-Step

The Bronchoscopy Step-by-Step© exercises were inspired by Arthur Murray's dance education principles. The most complex dance sequences, when broken down into numbered steps, can be learned step-by-step. Gradually, the steps are combined, and the moves finessed, until an elegant dance can be performed. Bach's thirty Goldberg variations are some of the most difficult to master pieces written for harpsichord and piano. No pianist learns them simultaneously; but with patience and guided focused practice, they can be mastered note by note by note. To cite another example, in becoming a good tennis player, one cannot master the forehand, backhand, serve, volley, smash and all other strokes at the same time; separately and repeatedly; however, these different strokes are practiced and then combined to play a beautiful game. It is noteworthy that as previously acquired habits are discarded and new approaches to the game or its techniques are acquired, learners are uncomfortable, and even resistant; their game might actually deteriorate until the new techniques become habit, and new muscle memory is acquired. The same holds true for bronchoscopy.

What these examples have in common is:

1. *Systematic Approach:* Deconstructing complex tasks into constituent elements
2. *Development of Muscle Memory:* Motor learning through the sub-conscious process of improving motor skills, smoothness and accuracy of movements, thus creating maximum efficiency and economy of movement. The major prerequisite for development of muscle memory is *repeated, deliberate practice.*
3. *Development of Spatial Awareness:* To learn to flow in space, always occupying the desired position. In bronchoscopy, this additionally requires the accurate identification of airway anatomy, and systematic exploration of lobar and segmental airways. For this Decision-Intention-Control are practiced in the context of Economy of Movement.

Remember: Decision; Intent; Control; Confidence; Economy of Movement.

All exercises are performed while observing basic principles. Optimum hand position and posture should be maintained at all times. The bronchoscope should be kept midline, minimizing white-out and red-out. The airway wall should be respected and trauma avoided. Steps should be practiced while standing both at the "patient's" head and side. It is best that exercises be practiced initially on inanimate models and/or a virtual reality (VR) simulator.

- **For instructional videos of these Bronchoscopy step-by-step go to:**
  Bronchoscopy Lessons. A series of lessons pertaining to aspects of bronchoscopy. http://www.youtube.com/watch?v=phRv73Ik7fI&feature=related. Search You Tube Bronchoscopy International (BronchOrg site).
- A poster of Bronchoscopy step-by-step exercises can be downloaded from www.Bronchoscopy.org
- Instructional videos and a poster handout are usually provided as part of training materials at regional Introduction to Flexible Bronchoscopy programs.

Bronchoscopy Step-by-Step

Step 1: Practice advancing from the nares or oral cavity (through a bite block) to the larynx. Identify structures as you proceed: nasal turbinates, hard and soft palate, uvula, posterior tongue, valeculla, epiglottis and frenulum, ariepylglottic folds and arythenoid cartilages, false and true vocal cords separated by the vestibule. Assess the movement and symmetry of the vocal cords upon tidal and deep respiration and phonation.

Step 2: Practice delivery of topical anesthetic (lidocaine) in small 1-2 ml. aliquots until anesthesia has been achieved. Observing the timing of breathing, during maximum abduction of the vocal cords, proceed beyond the vocal cords into the subglottic space (the widest point is usually near the posterior commissure). Examine the subglottic space while passing through the subgottic funnel, beyond the thyroid and cricoids cartilages, and first tracheal ring. Stopping in the subglottis is uncomfortable, induces cough and should be avoided unless absolutely necessary.

Step 3: Navigate from the subglottis, following the tracheal curve, to the carina. Then return to the subglottis. Repeat this exercise several times to master the small modifications necessary for rotation and flexion/extention of the distal tip of the bronchoscope that keeps the scope in the midline.

Step 4: Turn from the neutral position at the carina to the left, then back to the neutral position. Repeat many times. Then, turn from the neutral position at the carina to the right, then back to the neutral position. Repeat many times. Then practice doing each exercise both possible ways ("forward" and backward"). Then do the two exercises intermittently, one to the left, then to the right, then to the left, and so on. Then shuffle the exercises randomly, left and right and forward and backward.

Step 5: Turn from the neutral position at the carina to the left, down to the end of the LMB, and back up to neutral position at the carina. Do this exercise both possible ways ("forward" and backward"). Repeat many times. Then, turn from the neutral position at the carina to the right, down to the end of the RMB, then down the bronchus intermedius (BI), and return to neutral position at the carina. Do this exercise both possible ways ("forward" and backward"). Repeat many times. Then do the two exercises intermittently, one to the left, then to the right, then to the left, and so on. Then shuffle the exercises randomly, left and right and forward and backward.

Step 6: From the carina, follow the LMB, entering the two lobar bronchi (LLL and LUL) and return to the LMB and carina. Repeat several times. Then, from the carina, follow the RMB and BI, entering the three lobar bronchi (RML, RLL, and RUL) and return back to the RMB and carina. Repeat several times.

Steps 7 & 8: On the left, from the LMB, enter the LLL, first the Sup segment, then the basilar pyramid (Ant, Lat, Post). Then, from the LMB, enter the LUL, then each of the two divisions (Upper Div and Lingula), then each segment (Ant, Apical-Post, Sup-Ling, Inf-Ling). Then, perform the B-4-5-6 exercise, entering the Sup and Inf segments of the Lingula, followed by the Sup segment of the LLL.

On the right, from the RMB, follow the BI to the RML, and enter both segments of the RML (Lateral and Medial). Then, enter the RLL, first the Superior segment, then the basilar pyramid (Med, Ant, Lat, Post). Then, perform the B-4-5-6 exercise, entering the lateral and Medial segments of the RML, followed by the Superior segment of the RLL. Follow the Bronchus Intermedius and enter the RUL, entering all three segments (Ant, Post, Apical). Shuffle left and right exercises.

You are now ready to perform a complete inspection flexible bronchoscopy. Remember, there is usually no need to enter a segment more than once!

SECTION 4

Simulation Workshops

A series of *simulation workshops* and role-playing exercises include:

- *Informed consent- Patient safety* (includes universal, droplet, and airborne pathogens precautions) and *Procedural pause.*
- *Flexible bronchoscopy inspection with BAL, biopsy and brushing,* using inanimate models and/or high-fidelity computer-based virtual reality simulator.
- *Flexible bronchoscopy with TBLB and/or TBNA simulation,* using inanimate models and/or high-fidelity computer-based virtual reality simulator.

USER INSTRUCTIONS

Simulation Workshops

The purpose of these workshops is for learners to practice skills pertaining to flexible bronchoscopy without endangering or causing undue emotional or physical discomfort to patients. Using a combination of patient models, affordable low-fidelity case-based simulation, computer-based high-fidelity simulation, and interactive discussions and debriefing sessions, trainees and instructors work together to build a mutually productive educational environment consistent with the needs outlined in the ACGME Outcome Project.

Various assessment tools and *ten-point checklists* are used to document knowledge and skill acquisition in accordance with the elements required by ACGME (patient care, medical knowledge, practice-based learning and improvement, interpersonal communication skills, professionalism, and systems-based practice).

Case-based scenarios can be created by each training program, or scenarios already developed and tested can be used (some are downloadable from the Bronchoscopy.org website). Airway models, many of which are already being used internationally, can be purchased from organizations such as the American Association for Bronchology and Interventional Pulmonology and the Foundation for the Advancement of Medicine a (501-C3 nonprofit organization), as well as from private companies. Some can be loaned to institutions for specific courses.

Examples of Simulation Models

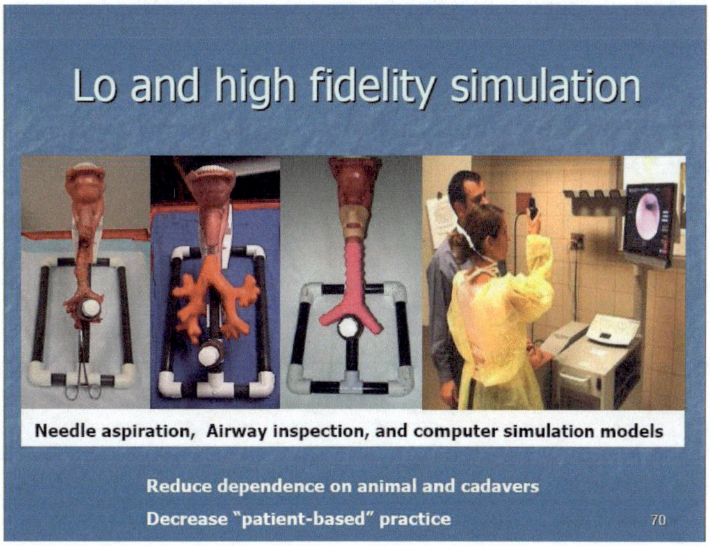

Informed Consent, Patient safety, and Procedural pause

Suggested learning materials (Items 1-6 should be reviewed prior to workshop participation)

1. Informed consent/research and procedures: read the essay from The Picture of Health: Medical ethics and the movies (Oxford University Press). View film clip from *Extreme Measures.*

2. Informed consent/competence and capacity: read the essay from The Picture of Health: Medical ethics and the movies (Oxford University Press). View film clip from *A Beautiful Mind.*

3. Simulation session: read case descriptions, debriefing and concepts.

4. Read the manuscript *Psychological Aspects of Flexible Bronchoscopy* (by Colt, Goldman, Edell, et al, available on Bronchoscopy.org).

5. Read *Medical Informed Consent: general considerations for physicians* (by Patrick et al).

6. Read the text abstracted from *Institute for Clinical Systems Improvement* (ICSI) *Guidelines for safe site invasive procedures non-operating room,* downloaded from http://www.icsi.org/ January 2010.

7. Read the text abstracted from Center for Disease Control *CDC Universal Precautions* downloaded from cdc.gov January 2010.

8. Participation in group session simulation workshop (duration 90 minutes) during which materials are reviewed and case-based simulations pertaining to informed consent, patient safety, and procedural pause are performed.

9. Interactive session with critical review of scene from the film *Death of Mr. Lazarescu.*

10. Interactive session (one-on-one assessment) with instructor for scoring and feedback purposes.

Informed Consent, Patient Safety, and Procedural Pause (Time-Out)*

Case Information

Part 1: Demographics

Case Title: Informed Consent, Patient Safety, Procedural Pause (Time Out)
Subject Name: (1) JL (2) BW (3) JJ
Scenario Name: Informed consent-patient safety-procedural pause
Simulation Developer(s): H. Colt
Date(s) of Development: January 2010

Appropriate for following learning groups

Post graduate education
Residents
Specialties: Pulmonary Anesthesiology Surgery Critical Care
Medical Students

Simulated patients 3 scenarios

Scenario # 1: (10 minutes, with 10 minutes debriefing): Obtain informed consent for flexible bronchoscopy from patient's wife. The patient has suspected left main bronchial obstruction. He is intubated and mechanically ventilated.

Scenario # 2: (10 minutes, with 10 minutes debriefing): Identify important elements of history and physical in a patient with tracheal stenosis and stridor being evaluated for flexible bronchoscopy and possible subsequent referral for bronchoscopic intervention (dilation, laser, stent insertion) or open surgery.

* Template for Simulation Patient. Design Modified from original template by *Jeffrey M. Taekman, M.D, Duke University Simulation and Patient Safety Center*

Scenario # 3: (10 minutes with 10 minutes debriefing): Review all of the elements of a Procedural Pause (Time Out) for a patient with AIDS, hemoptysis, left upper lobe infiltrate and suspected infectious lung disease about to undergo flexible bronchoscopy with bronchoalveolar lavage, brushing and transbronchial biopsy of the left upper lobe.

Scenario description: The instructor will read the scenario to the team. A specially trained patient educator will be the subject of the simulation. A team member will be designated to lead the simulation, and together with other team members, the team will proceed to perform each of the scenarios with guidance and specific instruction from the instructor. It is assumed that approximately ten minutes will be devoted to each scenario, with 10 minutes for an instructor-led debriefing. The instructor may choose to perform a ten minutes debriefing after moving the team through each of the three scenarios.

Part 2: Curricular Information

Educational Rationale:

There has been little or no emphasis on methods for obtaining informed consent for interventional pulmonary procedures, including flexible bronchoscopy. We believe that developing and applying guidelines for informed consent is necessary in view of the increasing number and complexity of interventional procedures to ensure that specific information about each procedure, as well as benefits, potential complications, and alternatives are shared with the patient. In addition, in an environment that respects cultural diversity, this information should be shared in respect with patient-defined goals, values and priorities, including participation of family members, when desired or warranted, in the information sharing and decision-making process.

Morbidity and mortality from medical errors is a growing concern for the public, and for healthcare professionals. Patient safety has become of outmost importance, especially in regards to interventional pulmonary diagnostic and therapeutic procedures, where, at least in the United States, where the legal system does not consider interventional pulmonologists to be practicing potentially dangerous or life-threatening procedures. Patient safety also includes knowledge and performance of the procedural pause, now mandatory in the Unites States in both the bronchoscopy suite and the operating room theater. We believe that it is possible to implement greater patient safety measures if bronchoscopists were regularly informed and instructed about these patient safety practices.

Learning Objectives:

- The learner should be able to characterize the informed consent process according to accepted criteria
- The learner should be able to characterize the informed consent process in the setting of an emergency airway procedure where interaction is only possible with a family member.

- The learner should be able to identify specific questions while obtaining the patient's history that help to ensure patient safety.
- The learner should be able to enumerate the elements of a procedural pause and lead the bronchoscopy healthcare team in a "time-out."

Guided Study Questions:

- What are the key elements of informed consent?
- In respect for cultural diversity, what elements should be taken into consideration?
- What key elements of the patient history are important for enhancing patient safety during an interventional diagnostic or therapeutic pulmonary procedure?
- What are the key elements of the procedural pause? Why is such a "time out" necessary?

References (in addition to those provided for this session)

- Braddock CH et al, How doctors and patients discuss routine clinical decisions. J. Gen Intern Med 1997;12:339-345
- Etchells E et al. Patient safety in surgery: error detection and prevention. World J Surg 2003;27:936-942.
- Colt HG. Functional evaluation before and after interventional bronchoscopy. In, Interventional Bronchoscopy, Prog Resp Research 2000; 30:55-65, Karger Eds.
- Joint Commission for the Accreditation of Healthcare Organizations. National Patient Safety Goals, 2006.
- ICSI Guidelines safe site invasive procedures non-operating room. Available from http://www.guideline.gov/summary/summary.aspx?ss=15&doc_id=13702 from

Didactics:

- Not applicable

Assessment Instruments:

- Informed consent checklist
- Procedural pause checklist
- Patient safety and procedure-related precautions checklist

Part 3: Preparation

Monitors Required:

Not applicable

Other equipment required:

Not applicable

Time Duration

For each scenario

Set-up	5 minutes
Preparation	2 minutes
Simulation	10 minutes
Debrief	10 minutes

Part 4: Supporting Files (case scenario handouts)

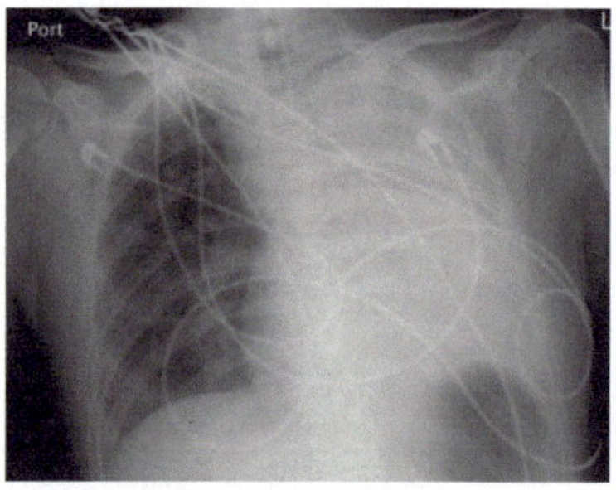

Scenario # 1 (Informed consent): A 60 year Korean old male with severe emphysema and a history of increasing shortness of breath, cough and weight loss has been hospitalized emergently with hypoxemia and respiratory failure. He is intubated and mechanically ventilated. Chest radiograph reveals opacification of the left hemithorax with ipsilateral shift of the mediastinum.

You must obtain informed consent from the patient's wife for flexible bronchoscopy in order to determine the cause for this radiographic finding.

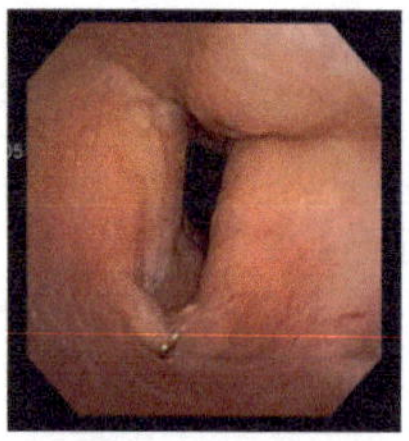

Scenario # 2 (Patient safety): A 42 year old African-American woman with increasing shortness of breath and a history of healed tracheotomy and severe rheumatoid arthritis is now admitted with stridor and cough. Three months earlier, bronchoscopy had revealed airway narrowing but the patient chose to do nothing.

In addition to obtaining informed consent, you must identify elements from the history that will help assure patient safety during and after the procedure.

Scenario # 3 (Procedural pause): A 30 year old male patient with AIDS, hemoptysis, left upper lobe infiltrate and suspected infectious lung disease is about to undergo flexible bronchoscopy with bronchoalveolar lavage, brushing and transbronchial biopsy of the left upper lobe.

In addition to the procedural pause, you must identify procedure-related elements such as universal precautions, droplet precautions, and airborne pathogen precautions instituted, before, during and after the procedure.

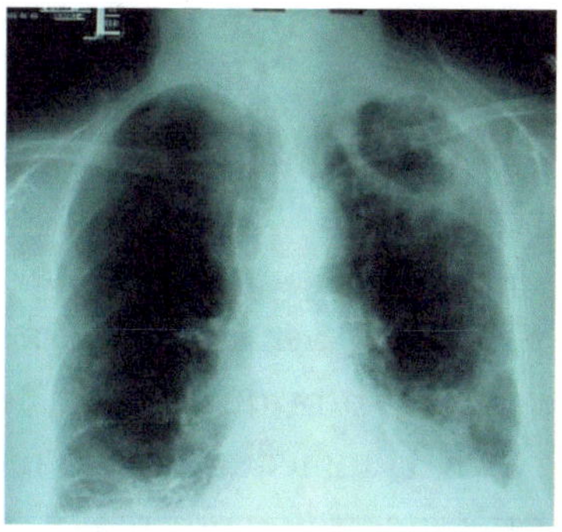

Part 5: Debriefing[1]

Scenario # 1: Informed Consent

Elements of informed decision making include: (1) discussion of the clinical issue, (2) description of the procedure, (3) discussion of risks and potential benefits of the procedure, (4) discussion of therapeutic alternatives and potential consequences from choosing those alternatives, (5) discussion of the implications of declining treatment, (6) assessment of the patient's and/or family member's understanding, (7) discussion of uncertainties associated with the decision, and (8) asking patient and family to express a preference.

Scenario # 2: Patient Safety and Precautions

Elements crucial to safe bronchoscopic intervention and follow-up include (1) review of medical history such as COPD, pulmonary embolus, deep venous thrombosis, rheumatoid arthritis, ankylosing spondylitis , infectious lung disease, other illnesses potentially affecting the airway, cardiac disease, pacemaker, coronary artery disease, obstructive sleep apnea, CO2 retention, laryngospasm or bronchospasm, asthma; (2) review of surgical history such as neck surgery, lung surgery, spine surgery; (3) dentures or loose teeth that might interfere with appropriate response to procedure-related complications; (4) bleeding disorder; (5) allergies to medications including local anesthetics, antibiotics, or reactions to general anesthetic drugs; (6) medication usage including anticoagulation, antiplatelet agents or clopidogrel (Plavix); (7) living situation and family or friend support system; (8) proximity to medical center and physician services; (9) pregnancy; (10) inquiry regarding advanced directives and health care decision making. (12) Universal precautions should always be used to protect the patient and the health care team from spread of blood borne infections such as Hepatitis and HIV. (13) Droplet precautions are warranted in case of risk for infectious lung disease which are droplet-transmitted (14) Airborne pathogens precautions are warranted in selected cases, especially in case of suspicion for tuberculosis or influenza. (15) Resuscitation cart must be readily available, a regularly checked and restocked.

[1] The reader is encourage to attend lectures pertaining to the above three subjects, in addition to reading the material provided in the real patient section of the training manual and reviewing the summary notes on the following pages.

Scenario # 3: Procedural Pause (Time-Out)

The procedural pause is performed immediately prior to the start of a procedure and must include specific elements to assure patient safety and avoid wrong procedure-wrong site-wrong patient events. A visual memory (triggers) is helpful to assure that all elements are addressed. These include (1) verification of patient, (2) verification of procedure, (3) verification of site and side, (4) verification of consistency with signed informed consent, (5) verification of availability of medical records and equipment, (6) declaration of need for medication or fluids, (7) description of allergies, drug reactions, (8) declaration and communication regarding other safety concerns. Initiated by the team leader, a verbal acknowledgement is required by all members of the health care team. During the time-out, each person in the room should stop what they are doing and actively participate in the process. No individual is exempt. Active participation requires that each individual state clearly that they agree with the elements of the time-out. Any discrepancies and disagreements must be addressed before the procedure is begun. If any distractions occur during the time-out, such as if another individual enters the room or a telephone rings, the time-out must be restarted.

Informed Consent Patient Safety and Time Out Slide Handout

INFORMED CONSENT

Bronchoscopy.org

Concept of Informed Consent

- Protects patient by providing information for informed decision-making
- Protects health care providers from liability provided procedure is executed according to prevailing standards and without negligence.
- Providers opportunity to consider and reconsider alternatives.
- Provides opportunity to discuss risks, benefits, and possible complications.

Bronchoscopy.org

Requirement for informed consent

- Must be informed and effective
- To be informed, a patient must be given information about the procedure relevant to their individual situation.
- To be effective, the person undergoing the procedure should be able to demonstrate in their own words, their understanding of the procedure or treatment.

Bronchoscopy.org

American Medical Association

- Informed consent is a "process" to discuss diagnosis and clinical issues
- As well as to discuss nature and purpose of proposed procedure., and its risks and benefits
- Discuss alternatives regardless of cost or insurance coverage, as well as potential risks and benefits of choosing an alternative
- Discuss risks and benefits of NOT receiving or undergoing the procedure.

Bronchoscopy.org

PATIENT SAFETY and PRECAUTIONS

Bronchoscopy.org

Universal Precautions

- Medical and surgical history, bleeding disorders, allergies, medications, pregnancy, living situation, proximity to physician services, advanced directives and medical decision-making.
- Universal precautions should always be used to protect the patient and the health care team from spread of blood borne infections such as Hepatitis and HIV.
- Gloves, Hand-washing, Gowns, Surface disinfection, Sharp containers

Bronchoscopy.org

Droplet precautions

- Droplet precautions are warranted in patients known or suspected to be infected with microorganisms transmitted by droplets (larger than 5 microns in size) that can be generated by coughing, sneezing, talking, or during the procedure.
  - Surgical masks, facial shield, or goggles
  - patient transport precautions
  - Droplet precaution sign on procedure room door
  - Cough/respiratory hygiene etiquette

Bronchoscopy.org

Airborne pathogens precautions

- Hand hygiene
- Cough/respiratory hygiene etiquette
- Cleaning and disinfection of contaminated surfaces
- Negative airflow with external exhaust
- N-95 respiratory or other National Institute for Occupational Safety and Health recommended device.
- Power air purifying respiratory (PAPR) might be considered in selected high risk cases.
- Airborne precautions sign

Bronchoscopy.org

PROCEDURAL PAUSE

Bronchoscopy.org

The concept of a "Procedural Pause", also known as a "Time Out"

- This safety protocol eliminates events involving the wrong patient, wrong site or wrong procedure.
- The protocol has been endorsed by more than fifty professional organizations, and is applicable to all high- risk procedures.
- The protocol is included in the USA Joint Commission for the Accreditation of Healthcare Organization National Patient Safety Goals project and was originally approved in 2004.
- The protocol also includes other components important in fostering a culture of patient safety, such as purposeful team communication and ensuring patient understanding.

Bronchoscopy.org

Requirements of an active "Time Out"

- Performed immediately prior to the start of the procedure.
- Ensures that the correct patient, site, positioning, and procedure to be performed are correctly identified.
- Ensures that pertinent imaging studies, medical records and equipment are available.
- Initiated by the provider and includes active verbal acknowledgement by all members of the health care team and any other persons present.
- All environmental distractions should be eliminated as much as possible.

Bronchoscopy.org

Time Out: visual memory guide

1. Verification of patient
   This is patient (read name badge), confirm with patient or family.
2. Verification of procedure "I am Dr.... We are going to perform ...Patient agrees..."
3. Verification of side and site
4. Nurse verifies consistency with signed informed consent.
5. Team members verify and declare availability of pertinent medical records, imaging studies and equipment.
6. Declare need for antibiotics, fluids or moderate sedation.
7. Describe allergies or drug reactions
8. Declare of safety issues based on medical history

Bronchoscopy.org

Excerpt from *Extreme Measures* & Informed Consent

The Picture of Health: Medical Ethics and Movies (Oxford University Press 2011)

Henri Colt M.D. FCCP (with permission)

Extreme Measures (1996). Hugh Grant, Gene Hackman, Sarah Jessica Parker. Directed by Michael Apted. Duration 120 minutes.

DVD Chapter 34 Scene 01:43:25 to 01:45:00

Extreme Measures tells the story of Dr. Guy Luthan (Hugh Grant), an Emergency Room physician entering a Neurology Fellowship in a New York Hospital. Luthan faces issues of conscience and professionalism after one of his patients, a homeless man with an identification wristband from a hospital Luthan has never heard of, dies and the body disappears. As he begins inquiries into the incident, he meets world-renowned Dr. Lawrence Myrick (Gene Hackman), a neurosurgeon who performs experimental spinal surgeries on the homeless in an attempt to find a cure to paralyzing spinal disorders.

In this scene, it appears that surgery has been performed without consent in physically fit, homeless individuals. The major protagonist of these actions. Dr. Myrick, declares that he is 68 years old, and does not have time to do experiments first in rats, then in chimpanzees. He further justifies human experimentation in nonconsenting, uninformed individuals by saying that great advances in medical science can only occur when physicians do what they think is right, even if it involves breaking rules. "People die everyday", he says, "And for what? For nothing. What do we do. What do you do? You take care of the ones you think you can save. Good doctors do the correct thing, but great doctors have the guts to do the right thing".

I often use the plot lines of *Extreme Measures* as springboards for discussions about informed consent, and more recently, about the appropriateness of incorporating a "time out" prior to any surgical intervention in order to help avoid performing inappropriate surgeries or operating on the wrong patient. With respect first to the surgery without consent issue, one needs to understand the legal notions of assault and battery. These were highlighted in the landmark case of *Schloendorff v Society of New York* regarding a surgeon who had performed a hysterectomy without consent. The law, which is based on the principle of self-determination[1], states that a person has the right to remain free from aggression against one's person.

From a legal perspective, *Assault* consists of a bodily threat and ability to do harm without a person's consent. Certainly, a surgeon has the ability to do harm either by operating inappropriately on a consenting patient, by performing procedures on a nonconsenting patient, and by performing the wrong procedure. Health care providers might also threaten to do harm by insisting on the performance of a procedure against a patient's wishes. *Battery,* on the other-hand, consists of any intentional bodily contact that violates the personal physical security of another without that person's permission. The batter victim does not need to be aware that physical violation has occurred. Such a scenario would apply to a patient who has been sedated or rendered unconscious by anesthesia. Nor do battery charges require that actual damage be demonstrated.

From a historical perspective, the doctrine of informed consent seems to have derived from the 1947 Nuremberg Code. This required doctors to obtain voluntary informed consent prior to conducting medical experimentation, and declared that all relevant information about a proposed procedure or treatment be provided prior to obtaining such consent. As a result of the Nuremberg trials, where it was discovered that Nazi doctors had performed grotesque medical experiments on prisoners and work camp detainees, Human Subjects Institutional Review Boards (IRBs) were created, in part to protect the rights of both patients and research subjects. With the World Medical Association's Declaration of Helsinki in 1964, an international code of ethics was also formulated to address concerns about the preservation of autonomy, beneficence, nonmaleficence, and justice for all human research subjects[2].

Institutional Review Boards (IRBs) oversee research protocols, monitor drug and treatment trials, and help investigators maintain appropriate records in case of inquiry[3]. In the United States, the Code of Federal Regulations Protection of Human Subjects (45CFR Part 46), is actually a direct result of various abuses of patient rights, such as those that occurred during the 30-year government-sponsored Tuskegee syphilis study, during which 300 black men were untreated despite the recognized effectiveness of antibiotic treatment. Today, one of an Institutional Review Board's major roles is, in fact, to assure that informed consent documents are written in such a way that all potential research subjects are able to understand the risks and benefits of any proposed research[4].

The American Medical Association has opinioned, however, that informed consent entails more than just informing patents about the risks and benefits of a proposed intervention or research project. It is a process of communication between a patient and a physician that results in the patient's authorization and agreement to undergo a specific medical intervention, ensuring that the patient has truly understood the elements of the procedure, as well as the consequences of undergoing or refusing to undergo the intervention[5]. It follows that physicians must disclose any and all conflicts of interest or compensation gained from any treatments or research being proposed. Similar recommendations have been issued by the British Medical Association, with emphasis on a patient-centered model of care whereby physicians are encouraged to take into consideration a patient's goals, values, and objectives and to provide information accordingly[6,7].

While the Nuremberg Code insisted on consent from research subjects, subsequent arguments have been made that in the case of therapeutic procedures on incompetent patients, and in research patients for whom there are no effective therapies, a strict requirement for informed consent may be viewed as contrary to the subject's best interests. Obviously, this argument cannot and should not be made in relation to this film, because the subjects of the experimental research in *Extreme Measures* are neither incompetent, nor are they the persons with disease. The film thus prompts one to ask whether the research might have been justified if it were being performed on those individuals with neurological injuries, rather than on the unwilling, disenfranchised, healthy, homeless subjects. Considering the ethical principles of autonomy, nonmaleficence, and a health care provider's duty to obtain informed consent, the answer to this question is a resounding no.

Regardless of place or type of medical practice, respect for individual autonomy mandates the informed consent process. Whether health care interventions occur from within a patient-focused or family-focused care model, informed consent is representative of shared decision making. Informed consent, as well as recently mandated surgical "time out" rules, helps ensure the satisfaction of legal and ethical obligations, and enhance the quality and safety of patient treatments and procedures[8].

In addition, the health care provider's duties to do no harm reasonably trump any arguments that might be presented to justify assault and battery in the clinical setting. In cases where there is a need for emergency intervention in incompetent patients, or in cases where patients are without decision making capacity and surrogate consent cannot be obtained, however, procedures might be performed on condition that patients could potentially benefit and that patient acceptance would be probable.

In *Extreme Measures*, however, justifications for performing surgery on individuals without their consent include the necessity to proceed with human experimentation because the results would benefit paralyzed patients. Another way to ponder some of the ethical dilemmas facing the health care providers in the film, as well as their administrative staff, therefore, is to reflect whether a common good (beneficence for society, or, in this case, specifically to the spinal disorders patient community), might in fact, warrant the physical, emotional, and psychological harm done to the unwilling study subject. This is counter, of course, to the principles of respect for autonomy and need to provide medical care while safeguarding a patient's best interests.

On the other hand, from a simple philosophical utilitarian perspective, one might argue that a greater good is accomplished for society as a whole, and that the disenfranchised study subjects provide no benefit to society other than their availability as objects of experimentation. If such an argument is deemed unacceptable, it is curious that similar perspectives are proposed to help justify the use and abuse of animals in research and procedural-based education, or the ready accessibility to patients, rather than to more costly inanimate and computer-based simulation in order to help health care providers improve their diagnostic and therapeutic procedural technical skills. In *Extreme Measures*, Myrick tells Luthan that the homeless persons undergoing experimental surgical procedures without consent, are, in fact, heroes because losing one to save millions is worthy of their sacrifice.

References

1. James L. Bernat, Lynn M. Peterson," Patient-centered informed consent in surgical practice," *Arch Surg* 141 (2006):86-92.
2. Declaration of Helsinki. Downloaded from http://www.wma.net/e/policy/b3.htm. Accessed, (November 20, 2008).
3. Robert A. Greenwald, Mary Kay Ryan, James E Mulvihill, *Human subjects research: A handbook for institutional review boards* (New York: Plenum Press, 1982).
4. Henri G. Colt, Ruth A Mulnard," Writing for a Human Subjects Institutional Review Board," *Chest* 130 (2006):1605-1607.

5. Council on Ethical and Judicial Affairs, *American Medical Association Code of Ethics,* 1st ed. (Chicago: American Medical Association, 2008)
6. Len Doyal, Jeffrey S. Tobias, eds. "Informed consent in medical research," *BMJ* 316 (March 28, 1998): 1000-5
7. John Bridson, Clare Hammond, Austin Leach, Michael R. Chester," Making consent patient centered," *BMJ* 327 (November 15, 2003):1159-1161.
8. Jessica W. Berg, Paul S. Appelbaum, *Informed consent: legal theory and clinical practice,* 2nd ed. (New York: Oxford University Press Inc, 2001).

Excerpt from *A Beautiful Mind* & Informed Consent

The Picture of Health: Medical Ethics and Movies (Oxford University Press 2011)

Jay A. Jacobson, M.D., MACP (with permission)

A Beautiful Mind (2001). Russell Crowe, Jennifer Connelly, Christopher Plummer
Directed by Ron Howard. Duration: 136 minutes

DVD chapter 16, Scene 01.39.05 to 01.42.30

A Beautiful Mind, inspired by a true story, explores the life, real and imagined, of John Nash Jr. (Russell Crowe) who is a brilliant, ultimately Nobel Prize winning mathematician, but who develops schizophrenia. His mind, still beautiful, but now untrustworthy, is capable of solving even previously insoluble theoretical problems, but is not always capable of distinguishing reality from paranoid delusions and visual and auditory hallucinations. His medical treatment consisted of insulin shock treatments and an orally administered drug, both accompanied by significant adverse effects. The drug, however, was somewhat effective in controlling the symptoms of schizophrenia. Based on a delusional preoccupation with a conspiracy and his negative experience with treatment, Nash subsequently rejects treatment which leads to nearly catastrophic consequences. Ultimately, forced or, at least, coerced treatment and his heroic will and capacity to compartmentalize and separate reality from fantasy enable Professor Nash to pursue his passion for mathematics, manage his life and relationships, and do the complex work that eventually earns him international acclaim.

On a windy morning when John is responsible for bathing their baby, his wife, Alicia (Jennifer Connelly) steps outside to bring in clothes hanging on the line. The sound of a radio and a banging door draw her to the shed where she is shocked by evidence of John's unabated schizophrenic delusions. Realizing that he is not taking his drug and fearful for the baby's safety, she rushes back inside the house, finds and rescues the frightened, crying baby from a tub rapidly filling with water. Actively hallucinating, John imagines that his wife's call to his doctor constitutes a threat and knocks her down with their baby.

In the critical scene, Dr. Rosen has come to the Nash home. John admits that he stopped his medicine because of its side effects and he acknowledges persistent visual hallucinations. Dr. Rosen warns him that, if untreated, schizophrenia will only worsen and he recommends readmission to the hospital for more insulin shock and drug therapy. John is reluctant to begin another traumatic hospitalization that he fears will never end. Dr. Rosen has commitment papers which Alicia can sign that mandate admission and treatment. John hopes that she won't sign and wishes for more time to work this problem out. He affirms the doctor's judgment that "I'm not safe anymore". When Alicia asks him if he would hurt her, he says, "I don't know".

This scene illustrates the problem posed by the multi-tiered concept of informed consent, especially in the context of mental illness where decision making capacity and competence are especially hard to isolate and evaluate. The policy and practice of voluntary informed consent arose in response to forced, experimental and even lethal treatment of prisoners in Nazi concentration camps. We follow this practice in clinical settings as well. We grant patients with the mental capacity to make decisions a near absolute right to do so. We expect physicians to provide ample information and permit unforced consent or refusal. They should explain the indications for a treatment, its risks and benefits and the comparative results of treatment, alternative treatment, and no treatment.

One prerequisite for voluntary informed consent is an environment free of a compelling force that will drive the decision in one direction and negate the patient's ability and freedom to choose. Another is the mental capacity to make a reasoned choice. One way to assess this capacity is to establish if the patient has a set of values and goals, if the patient can communicate and understand information and can reason and deliberate about the choice.

In this scene, we have a physician who makes an assessment and recommends the medically indicated treatment. He predicts what will happen without treatment. He doesn't address side effects, but also does not dispute the observations that John makes about the negative effects of drug treatment. John has prior personal experience with the risks and benefits of treatment. Thus, to some extent the "informed" criteria for voluntary informed consent are met. What remains to be considered is whether John Nash, with his undeniable mental capacity for mathematical problem solving, has the mental capacity to make a reasonable and uncoerced personal treatment decision. If he lacks this capacity, others with his best interest in mind, can and should make the choice for him. If he has the capacity and refuses the therapy that others think best for him are there valid and ethical reasons to override that choice?

John, even in his unmedicated, self acknowledged delusional state does seem to have sustained values and goals. His goal is to pursue his professional work, to solve problems. He values knowledge and his emotional attachment to his wife and child. He is able to communicate and understand information from the doctor, although he reaches a different conclusion about treatment. Unfortunately, we've seen that he can't reliably discriminate between information coming from a real or an imagined source. He does seem to be able to reason about and give reasons for his choices. His belief about the result of another hospitalization demonstrates his ability to connect an intervention with an outcome even if the outcome he foresees may not be the positive one that the doctor and Alicia are hoping for. It is a possible and plausible outcome.

A person's ability to make decisions is both ethically and legally important. In law, it permits individuals to make choices, even those judged unwise by others, and it makes individuals responsible for intentional actions that break laws or harm others. In medical ethics, it is the basis for providing relevant information to patients prior to treatment or procedures and for respecting their decision to proceed or refuse. Legal cases about cognitive ability often arise in the context of financial matters, reproductive choices or crimes. Medical ethics discussions of this ability usually pertain to decisions that affect the individual's health. The law presumes that individuals acquire sufficient decision making ability when they become adults. The age of adulthood, rather than some demonstrated ability, becomes the standard and is set by statute. The law regards adults, absent evidence to the contrary, to be able and entitled to make their own decisions. The legal term for this is competent. Adults retain the right to make a full range of decisions for themselves unless a judge rules, based on evidence, that they are incompetent. Medical ethics is attentive to context and to individual differences in ability. In emergencies, for example, when medical decisions must be made quickly, if patients are temporarily mentally impaired or even unconscious, physicians generally proceed with treatment despite their patient's impaired or absent decision making capacity. This is justified by the concept of implied consent.

When an adult patient's condition is not emergent and life threatening the law and medical ethics agree that consent for treatment is imperative. For patients who are obviously and permanently impaired who don't refuse treatment, physicians turn to family members to make the decision they believe the patient would have made or, if that's unknown, the decision that would be best for the patient. When patients, who have been functioning independently and making their own decisions, refuse treatment for a dangerous and serious condition, doctors and concerned family members understandably question the patient's ability and right to make what seems to them to be an irrational and self destructive decision. Before they can force an expressly unwanted medical intervention, physicians should attempt to understand the patient's reasons and capacity to make such decisions.

This medical assessment could be as simple as asking the patient five questions: What is the medical problem? What treatment has been recommended? What will happen to you with and without the treatment? Finally, what is the reason for the decision? Patients with decision making capacity demonstrate a correct understanding of the nature of the medical problem, its treatment and prognosis, and have a reason for the decision. When such patients offer a reason that seems irrational and unconnected with a personal, religious, or cultural set of beliefs and values, a more expert evaluation by a mental health professional is appropriate. The expert may conclude that the patient, even though mentally or emotionally ill, has the capacity to make medical decisions. If this expert decides the patient lacks decision making capacity, the patient or someone on his behalf may still assert his legal competence and right to refuse treatment. If the patient appears to be a threat to himself or others, clinicians can temporarily take steps such as hospitalization to address that danger. However, to continue this beyond two or three days or begin treatment will require that a legal determination of competence be made.

Based on her questions to the patient, information from the family, and the opinion of experts, a judge decides whether a patient is competent. If so, the patient retains his right to refuse treatment. If not, the judge will appoint someone to be the guardian and decision maker for the patient. This could be a family member or someone specifically chosen for this task.

The film, *A Beautiful Mind*, doesn't include a legal determination of competence and it is ambiguous about whether John Nash is ultimately persuaded or voluntarily chooses medical treatment. Fortunately for him and for the viewers he somehow becomes able to manage the symptoms of his mental illness and resume a meaningful professional and family role. A patient's mental illness and impaired decision making often cause physicians and family members to feel frustration as they try to do what they believe is best for patients, but encounter what they view as legal obstacles. The law, however, is there to safeguard competent patients' rights and protect their liberty to make even seemingly unwise decisions. The law does balance the rights of individuals to decide against the consequences of their decision for others. Interestingly, even competent patients may have their liberty curtailed if they refuse treatment for a readily communicated serious disease such as tuberculosis. Thus, imminent danger to others and self is a reason for hospitalization or institutionalization that doctors, families, and judges can all agree on.

When diseases are dire and their treatments are safe, simple, well tolerated, inexpensive, highly effective and life saving, doctors zealously advocate for them and most patients accept their recommendation. When we develop fully effective, better tolerated treatments for mental illnesses such as schizophrenia, patients may be more willing to accept them and thus help us avoid the ethically, legally, and emotionally fraught decision to force treatment.

References

1. Applebaum PS. Assessment of patients' competence to consent to treatment. *N Engl J Med 2007*; 357:1834-1840.
2. Brock DW, Wartman SA. When competent patients make irrational choices. *N Engl J Med* 1990;323:1353-1355.
3. Grisso T, Appelbaum PS. *Assessing Competence to Consent to Treatment: A Guide for Physicians and Other Health Professionals*. NY, NY. Oxford University Press, 1998.
4. Kim SYH. When does decisional impairment become decisional incompetence? Ethical and methodological issues in capacity research in schizophrenia. *Schizophr Bull* 2006;32:92-97.
5. President's Commission for the Study of Ethical Problems in Medicine and Biomedical and Behavioral Research. *Making health care decisions*: a report on the ethical and legal implications of informed consent in the patient practitioner relationship. Vol 1. Washington, DC: Government Printing Office, 1982.

SECTION 5

Observed Real-Patient Scenarios

A series of *observed real-patient scenarios** that include:

- An *informed consent, patient safety, procedural pause* scenario.
- A *flexible bronchoscopy inspection with BAL, brushing and biopsy* scenario.
- A *flexible bronchoscopy with TBLB and/or TBNA* scenario.

* Checklists and assessment tools used at the discretion of program director.

USER INSTRUCTIONS

Real patient observations

The purpose of real patient observations is to allow the instructor to assess the learner in the clinical setting. This is similar to how medical students and other house officers are observed and judged prior to being deemed competent to perform a physical examination or certain procedures.

Various assessment tools and ten-point checklists are used to document knowledge and skill acquisition in accordance with elements required by ACGME (patient care, medical knowledge, practice-based learning and improvement, interpersonal communication skills, professionalism, and systems-based practice).

It is assumed that learners will be observed throughout their subspecialty training, and that specific instances may be chosen for assessment purposes. The frequency of such assessments is still undetermined, but the purpose is to be able to monitor the learner's progression along the learning curve, so that instructors might be able to provide constructive feedback and advice, in addition to knowledge and technical expertise.

Learners are encouraged to build on the knowledge gained from simulation sessions, and to read (1) The psychological aspects of flexible bronchoscopy and informed consent process, (2) The extract from Institute for Clinical Systems Improvement Guidelines for Time Out (procedural pause), and (3) The extract from the Center for Disease Control's guide on Universal precautions.

The learner may wish to keep a diary of procedures performed. An example of such a log is provided below.

Patient identification	Date of procedure	Procedures performed (inspection, biopsy, washings, BAL, Brushing, TBNA, TBLB)	Complications (None if applicable)	Results (includes response to complications and laboratory data)
1				
2				
3				
4				
5				

Procedure log

Bronchoscopist ____

Patient identification and Indication for procedure	Date of procedure	Procedures performed (Inspection, Biopsy, Washings, BAL, Brushing, TBNA, TBLB)* *Circle all those that apply	Complications (None if applicable)	Results (includes response to complications and laboratory data)
1		I, Bx, W, BAL, Br, TBNA, TBLB		
2		I, Bx, W, BAL, Br, TBNA, TBLB		
3		I, Bx, W, BAL, Br, TBNA, TBLB		
4		I, Bx, W, BAL, Br, TBNA, TBLB		
5		I, Bx, W, BAL, Br, TBNA, TBLB		
6		I, Bx, W, BAL, Br, TBNA, TBLB		
7		I, Bx, W, BAL, Br, TBNA, TBLB		
8		I, Bx, W, BAL, Br, TBNA, TBLB		
9		I, Bx, W, BAL, Br, TBNA, TBLB		
10		I, Bx, W, BAL, Br, TBNA, TBLB		
11		I, Bx, W, BAL, Br, TBNA, TBLB		
12		I, Bx, W, BAL, Br, TBNA, TBLB		
13		I, Bx, W, BAL, Br, TBNA, TBLB		
14		I, Bx, W, BAL, Br, TBNA, TBLB		
15		I, Bx, W, BAL, Br, TBNA, TBLB		
16		I, Bx, W, BAL, Br, TBNA, TBLB		
17		I, Bx, W, BAL, Br, TBNA, TBLB		
18		I, Bx, W, BAL, Br, TBNA, TBLB		
19		I, Bx, W, BAL, Br, TBNA, TBLB		
20		I, Bx, W, BAL, Br, TBNA, TBLB		
21		I, Bx, W, BAL, Br, TBNA, TBLB		
22		I, Bx, W, BAL, Br, TBNA, TBLB		
23		I, Bx, W, BAL, Br, TBNA, TBLB		
24		I, Bx, W, BAL, Br, TBNA, TBLB		
25		I, Bx, W, BAL, Br, TBNA, TBLB		
26		I, Bx, W, BAL, Br, TBNA, TBLB		
27		I, Bx, W, BAL, Br, TBNA, TBLB		
28		I, Bx, W, BAL, Br, TBNA, TBLB		
29		I, Bx, W, BAL, Br, TBNA, TBLB		
30		I, Bx, W, BAL, Br, TBNA, TBLB		

The psychological aspects of flexible bronchoscopy and the process of informed consent

Henri Colt, M.D., Alan J. Goldman, M.D., John Knippa, Ph.D and Eric Edell, M.D.

Introduction

In Carol Izard's *Psychology of Emotions*, "fear" is defined as "certain bodily changes, expressive behaviors, and feelings that result from the apprehension of threat or danger". It is a separate and distinct emotion, different from anxiety, which is described as an uneasy, apprehensive feeling caused by a combination or pattern of emotions, including fear, that affect social relationships, bodily states, perceptions, thoughts, and actions[1].

Both fear and anxiety are caused by invasive medical procedures. In this paper, we address specific causes of procedure-related emotional distress, summarize research findings in regards to bronchoscopy-related anxiety, describe the various elements of informed consent, and propose a strategy whereby health care providers might integrate the recognition and alleviation of procedure-related anxiety into the process of informed consent.

Procedure-related emotional distress is frequently based on a patient's belief that medical procedures will cause pain, disability, or even death. Feelings of anxiety and fear are often accompanied by a sensation of helplessness and loss of control, sometimes exacerbated by memories of emotional suffering, physical pain and even grief prompted by previous medical encounters. The person *with disease*, is after all, quite different from the same healthy person living prior to disease, and in the unfamiliar and often intimidating surroundings of a sterile procedure room, surrounded by strangers busily going about their business, many patients might even begin to think of themselves as *victims of* rather than as *participants in* their medical care.

While compassion, empathy, and reassurance are paramount to restoring a patient's emotional and psychological well being, the truth is that many health care providers are not sufficiently aware of, or trained to recognize the pre-procedural emotional turmoil that patients often experience. Hence, health care providers may not implement or actively participate in appropriate measures that assist in reducing procedure-related emotional distress. Furthermore, when health care providers "invade" the human body to treat or to obtain the vital tissue information that is necessary to secure a definitive diagnosis, they often focus on filling out their paperwork, preparing their instruments, discussing the case with colleagues and students present at the patient's bedside, and verifying the accuracy of patient-related data. All too often the emotional toll of invasive pain and anxiety-producing procedures on their patients is exacerbated, downplayed or forgotten.

Traditionally, information about the risks, benefits, potential alternatives and consequences of not undergoing a specific intervention or treatment is addressed during the informed consent process. The emotional distress related to illness, suspected diagnosis or procedure-related outcomes, however, is not easily addressed during this frequently brief patient-physician-family encounter. This is because a physician's focus is usually on obtaining authorization to proceed with a procedure rather than on using informed consent as an opportunity for dialogue.

In addition, not all practitioners have the knowledge, training or desire to recognize, address and alleviate an individual's emotional and psychological concerns. If the informed consent process is considered to be a burdensome exercise rather than an opportunity for communication, a patient's questions are often left unanswered, or worse still, left unsaid, such that a patient's concerns remain unaddressed. Not infrequently, consent is obtained almost mechanically, as part of something the physician must, rather than chooses, to do. Even in the best of cases, the tendency for physicians to unintentionally impose their values, opinions and feelings on a patient is difficult to avoid. Despite good intentions, many practitioners are insufficiently trained to recognize and respond effectively to a patient's psychological distress, which, like pain (now considered a vital sign), is not always overtly displayed.

During the process of true informed consent, professional caregivers, patients and family members have an opportunity for education, shared decision-making, and partnership. While recognition and relief of a patient's procedure-related anxieties and fears are possible through open communication, such a dialogue is not always easy to initiate or maintain because of cultural biases, lack of knowledge or understanding, and time restrictions on consultative medical practices. As the medical, legal, social, and ethical obligations of informed consent become increasingly apparent, physicians will need to master the art of empathic communication and learn to apply this skill to the informed consent process. Not surprisingly, the acquisition of communication and professionalism skills has, in the United States, become an integral part of the Accreditation Council of Graduate Medical Education guidelines for competency-based physician training[2].

Procedure-related fear and anxiety with a focus on bronchoscopy

Flexible bronchoscopy is a common medical procedure, with more than 500,000 studies being performed yearly by chest physicians in the United States alone[3]. It is frequently performed in an outpatient setting and allows physicians to visually evaluate the larynx, the trachea and the lower airways of the respiratory system. It is used diagnostically and therapeutically for viewing abnormalities of the airways, obtaining tissue specimens from the lungs, removing tracheal or bronchial foreign objects, resecting benign and malignant tumors, or for restoring airway patency.

Patients undergoing bronchoscopy often have life-threatening illnesses, suspected cancer, lung infections, airway obstruction, and symptoms of cough, shortness of breath, or hemoptysis. The procedure is usually completed in less than twenty minutes. It is usually considered safe regardless of whether it is performed in the awake, moderately sedated or anesthetized patient, although risks of oversedation, hypoxemia, respiratory insufficiency, pneumothorax and bleeding must be acknowledged[4]. Bronchoscopy can cause transient dysphagia, nose pain, and throat pain. Procedure-induced coughing, gagging, and shortness of breath further increase the discomfort and anxiety felt by an already apprehensive and possibly ill patient. Also present is the anxiety-producing possibility of an incomplete or non-diagnostic study that could necessitate repeating the procedure[5].

Procedure-related anxiety is, for the most part, a complex, subjective response thought to be influenced most importantly by a patient's temperament and understanding, or lack of understanding, of their illness and the proposed intervention. Excessive degrees of anxiety can lead to heightened physiological responses such as vasoconstriction, tachycardia, hypertension, and cardiac arrhythmias. In some patients, even the insertion of a simple intravenous catheter during the pre-procedure phase can become a difficult task as a result of anxiety-related peripheral vasoconstriction. In regards to flexible bronchoscopy, the standard of practice in most countries is to offer patients anti-anxiety medication[6].

Studies have shown that increased pre-procedure anxieties correlate most with increased post-procedure reports of pain, medication requirements, and prolonged post-procedure hospital stays. Desbiens et al.[7] reported that patients with greater anxiety and depression more often reported <u>less</u> satisfaction with pain control and hospitalization. Almost twenty years ago, Hicks and Jenkins[8] described a number of indirect objective measures of anxiety such as heart rate, blood pressure, degree of skin conductance, plasma cortical and catecholamine levels, and urinary catecholamine excretion levels that can become elevated in these pre-procedure anxiety states.

Since then, a number of publications have reported various medications or techniques that have attempted to reduce patients' anxieties and help make bronchoscopy and other invasive procedures go more smoothly and more quickly for both patients and physicians. Validated questionnaires such as the State-Trait Anxiety Inventory, the Amsterdam Pre-Operative & Information Scale questionnaire, and the Visual Analogue Scale have been used to assess a patient's pre-procedure psychological state in order to define, measure, and monitor a patient's emotional status[9-12]. Results from these studies have confirmed the frequent presence of procedure-related anxiety, and highlighted the difficulties practitioners often encounter in relieving emotional and psychological concerns.

Pre-procedure techniques to reduce patient anxieties have included the use of simple explanatory brochures or videotapes about the procedure, informed consent forms that further describe details of the procedure and its related potential adverse events, allowing the patient to walk into the procedure room instead of being wheeled into the theater on a gurney[13], distraction therapy using nature scene murals or nature sounds[14], music[15-19], guided imagery[20], conscious sedation[21], visitor contact[22], stress inoculation[23] and hypnosis[24].

These techniques, including the administration of stronger or longer lasting pre-procedure anesthetic and amnestic agents, are aimed at reducing a patient's sense of anxiety caused by the "not knowing" what they will be experiencing. Most are based on the conscious distraction by the patient onto other thought processes and away from a focus on the upcoming procedure. Guided imagery, for example, uses the power of thought to influence psychological and physiologic states. Stress inoculation, on the other-hand, is a multi-step process that teaches individuals how to prepare for and actively cope with the stressors that they may incur during a medical procedure or treatment.

It appears that educating patients about the procedure appears to be the single most important and most easily manageable pre-procedure factor in lowering emotional concerns and procedure-related discomfort[25]. This is the case, even in individuals whose psychological profiles show them to have very low levels of underlying "Trait" personality anxieties. Such educational interventions might be ideally delivered during inpatient or outpatient consultation, rather than at the time of the procedure itself.

What is also apparent from the literature, is that there has been little or no emphasis placed on a having a uniform method of informed consent for bronchoscopy. The American Medical Association states that informed consent entails more than just informing patents about the risks and benefits of a proposed intervention. It is a process of communication between a physician and a patient that results in the patient's authorization and agreement to undergo a specific medical intervention, ensuring that the patient has truly understood the elements of the procedure, as well as the consequences of undergoing or refusing to undergo the intervention[26]. Similar recommendations have been issued by the British Medical Association, with emphasis on a patient-centered model of care whereby physicians are encouraged to enquire into and consider a patient's goals, values, and objectives, and to provide information accordingly[27]. Indeed, the informed consent process appears to provide an ideal opportunity for health care providers to recognize, address and alleviate a patient's fears and anxieties related to a procedure such as flexible bronchoscopy.

The Process of Informed Consent

The concept of *Voluntary Informed Consent* has been studied by the American judicial system for a number of years[28]. It is the legal embodiment of the concept that each individual has the right to make decisions affecting his or her well-being[29]. The "Doctrine of Informed Consent" may have been originally derived from the 1947 Nuremberg Code which required that doctors obtain the voluntary informed consent of a subject prior to conducting medical experimentation. As a result of these Nuremberg trials, where it was discovered that Nazi doctors had performed grotesque medical experiments on prisoners and work camp detainees, Human Subjects Institutional Review Boards and ethics committees were also created, in part to protect the rights of both patients and research subjects, and to assure compliance with the subsequent 1964 World Medical Association's Declaration of Helsinki formulation of an international code of ethics to address concerns about the preservation of autonomy, beneficence, nonmaleficence, and justice for all human research subjects[30].

The Informed Consent Doctrine requires that medical doctors provide a patient with all relevant information about a proposed procedure or treatment prior to obtaining the consent of the patient to carry out that procedure or treatment. Informed consent protects the patient by providing them with complete information on which to make an informed decision. Informed consent may also, at times, protect the health care provider from liability (with exceptions) provided that the procedure is properly executed according to the prevailing standards of care in the community and without negligence. In addition, the informed consent process gives health care providers and patients an opportunity to consider and re-consider the diagnostic and therapeutic strategies being proposed, as well as the possible risks and benefits of such procedures and to prepare, as needed, for procedure-related adverse events. From a patient's perspective, one might prepare for and lessen procedure-related anxiety by designating surrogate decision makers in case of procedure-related complications, assuring notification about advanced directives and code status, or by requesting the presence of family members at the time of the intervention.

From a legal standpoint, at least in the United States, consent for a medical procedure must be both *informed* and *effective.* To be *informed,* a person must be given information about the procedure relevant to their individual situation. To be *effective,* the person undergoing the procedure should be able to demonstrate, in his or her own words, their understanding of the procedure. Merely asking a person if they understand and receiving a "yes" or a head nod in response is generally considered insufficient. In some countries, informed consent needs to be documented by signatures from patients, witnesses, and health care providers on a specially-designed document approved for use by the institution's medical and risk management committees. The validity in court of such documents has been debated, however, and in some North American institutions, physicians may be counseled to additionally describe the informed consent process in their dictated preprocedure notes.

Informed consent, therefore, is more than simply requesting that a patient sign a written consent form. It is a *process of communication* between a patient and a physician that results in the patient's authorization or agreement to undergo a specific medical intervention. During this dialogue, the physician who is performing the procedure; not a delegated representative, should disclose and discuss: (i) The patient's diagnosis, if known, or the concerning clinical issues, (ii) the nature and purpose of the proposed treatment or procedure, (iii) the risks and benefits of the proposed treatment or procedure (iv) alternative treatments regardless of their costs or if covered by health insurance, (v) potential risks and benefits from choosing alternative treatments or procedures, and (vi) the risks and benefits of <u>not</u> receiving or undergoing a treatment or procedure.

The patient in turn, should be given the opportunity to ask any questions which they deem necessary to gain a better understanding of the procedure so that an informed decision can be made to proceed with or to refuse that particular course of medical intervention. Health care providers should assure that the patient has truly understood the elements of the procedure as well as the elements of the informed consent process. This can be done by asking the patient to repeat, in their own words, their understanding of the procedure. From an ethics perspective, physicians should be expected to disclose any conflicts of interest or compensation gained from the treatments or procedures performed[31].

In children (when a patient is under 18 years of age, unless married or otherwise considered to be an "emancipated minor") or if an adult patient is mentally or physically incompetent, incapacitated, or if no Health Care Directive exists, a parent or other guardian can usually give surrogate consent or "permission", assuming that the surrogate has decisional capacity and legal empowerment to give such consent for medical care and that the surrogate is acting with the patient's best interest in mind and according to what the patient would have wanted had the patient been able to participate in the decision-making process. In the United States, when there is no guardian, the provisions of Section 59 of the Guardianship and Administration Act of 1993 apply and consent must then be obtained from a spouse, including a legal de-facto spouse, a parent, a sibling over 18 years of age, a son or daughter over 18 years of age, or a person (not being the guardian) who acts *in loco parentis.*

In emergency situations, a physician can proceed without obtaining consent when treatment is needed urgently to save a person's life or to prevent serious damage to a person's health and (i) the treating health care provider does not have any knowledge of a prior refusal by the person to the treatment, (ii) the patient has not appointed a Medical Agent, (iii) the patient has not appointed an Enduring Guardian, and (iv) there is no Guardianship Order with a guardian appointed by a Guardianship Board. Surprisingly, there is often very little difference between consent forms used for elective versus emergency procedures. In some cases, the content of these forms does not even meet the accepted standards of information delivery[32]. In addition, during emergencies, attention is not often given to an individual's level of understanding of their illness or, in some cases, to that individual's ability to even read or truly comprehend the informed consent form that they are expected to sign[1].

Informed Consent, Capacity, Competence, and the Law

The informed consent process in the United States and in most other countries is designed to ensure not only the satisfaction of legal, ethical, and accreditation requirements, but also the *quality* and *safety* of patient treatments and procedures. A patient's right to informed consent or to refuse a medical treatment or procedure can thus be enforced in a number of ways, including through state common law, federal and state statutes and regulations, medical ethics, and Joint Commission hospital guidelines.

Studies outside of the realm of bronchoscopy have shown that even after consent is obtained, 18% to 45% of patients can not state the major risks associated with their procedures[33]. It is unclear whether this is the result of poor communication, lack of information, poor recall as a consequence of procedure-related stress and anxiety, or absence of memory reinforcement. At least one study has shown that patients who are simply asked to recount what they have learned during the informed consent discussion have greater recall and comprehension of that interaction than those who are not asked to recount the interaction[34]. A written and signed consent form, while not replacing the discussion between a patient and their provider, supports legal evidence such as testimony and notes in the medical record, of the validity of the patient's informed and agreed upon understandings and statements concerning the procedure.

Underlying the concept of informed consent is the assumption that a patient is cognitively competent. From the sociological standpoint, *competence* is defined as having sufficient ability to make choices such that personal autonomy remains intact. Legally, *competence* is a state in which an individual's decision-making ability is adequate to meet the demands of a clearly specified decision-making task. A person may therefore be competent in some endeavors but not in others. Based on a review of judicial opinions and case law in the United States, legal standards of competence to consent to procedures include the ability to understand the information that is provided, the ability to appreciate one's own situation in light of the information provided, the ability to reason with the information provided, and the ability to express a choice. Curiously, only the abilities to understand information and to express a choice are universally held as legal standards upon which to base a determination of competence[35].

Technically, medical professionals lack the legal authority to determine competence, and instead are able to determine whether a patient has decision-making *capacity*. A patient may, for example, be capable of making the decision to refuse to undergo a procedure, yet be found legally incompetent to handle their personal finances. Often, a physician's assessment of decision-making capacity guides legal determinations of competence, and it is frequently the physician's finding of incapacity that causes alternative forms of consent to be sought, and a patient's legal rights to be temporarily suspended without involvement of the courts.

It seems reasonable to question whether voluntary choice and decisional competence and capacity are truly preserved in a medical emergency. There are considerable barriers, conscious and unconscious, as well

[1] An excellent example of this is found in the 2005 Romanian film *The Death of Mr. Lazarescu* directed by Cristi Puiu.

as intellectual and emotional, to assimilating information during an acute illness, trauma, or life-threatening event. It is generally accepted that patients who have received sedatives or narcotics as part of a treatment plan for respiratory insufficiency, intubation, pain, or high-grade anxiety should not be asked for permission to perform invasive procedures.

Sometimes, even the stress of illness may suffice to alter the decision-making capacities of otherwise reasonable individuals. Studies of patients with acute myocardial infarctions, for example, suggest that psychological or physical stress alone may compromise understanding[36-38]. Assessments of decisional abilities before a determination of capacity can be reached are also difficult in patients with suspected neurologic or cognitive impairment accompanied by communicative dysfunction, especially when there is limited time in which to institute a treatment plan; for example, when emergency intubation is required for survival (note that as of this writing, there is no validated instrument for measuring cognitive and procedure-related decision-making capacity in patients with acute stroke).

Procedure-related anxiety and the informed consent process

A patient's emotions and psychology have considerable impact on the informed consent process. Aklad, et al[39], in a paper published in 2004, noted that current procedures for obtaining informed consent neither adequately reflect the patient's own views and values nor address their emotional and psychological needs in a time of probable increased vulnerability. Patients were noted to have felt frightened or under pressure at the time of the informed consent. They were significantly more likely to report procedure satisfaction if they saw a familiar face, such as one of their health care providers, prior to the procedure <u>and</u> if they received detailed information about their procedure from that same individual. Kondziolka et al[40] approached this issue by developing a procedure-based consent process that facilitated patient discussion. In their study, post- procedure interviews showed a high rate of patient recall of the procedure and of the consent discussions, as well as high satisfaction ratings for both the consent process and the procedure performed.

Race, ethnicity, gender, socio-economic status, education, a patient's previous experiences with physicians, and health care system culture, also impact a patient's emotional and psychological well-being in preparation for a procedure[41]. Hattori et al[42] and Ruhnke et al[43] reported that in Japan, family and physician opinions alone, rather than the patient's thoughts or concerns, are accorded a larger role in clinical decision making than in the United States. This may also be the case in other medical cultures. In Latin America, for instance, family-focused rather than patient-focused care seems to be a major determinant of medical decision making[44]. Regardless of medical environment and practice setting, the potentially coercive powers of family members, friends, other physicians, and ancillary health care providers capable of influencing a patient's decisions cannot be denied.

Obtaining proper informed consent and lowering a patient's procedure-related anxiety are not easily combined. Many written informed consent forms generically describe the *mechanics* of an invasive procedure, while any discussion regarding the *sensations* a patient might experience while undergoing the procedure is assumed to be initiated by the physician. Unlike pain and other vital signs, however, there is virtually no evidence of consideration for a patient's emotional state prior to an intervention.

The narcissistic wound of severe illness is real, although not always readily apparent. It is well recognized that illness changes a person's perception of oneself and of others, often also altering a person's traditional value system. This places patients in a position of weakness as compared to their empowered health care providers, family members, and previously empowered selves. Too much information, or information provided in an inappropriate fashion, potentially increases procedure-related anxiety. It is not surprising, therefore, that a review of thirty-four studies of disclosure techniques designed to *improve patient understanding* found that better understanding correlates with highly structured oral presentations that make use of visual illustrations, simplified written consent forms, and brief summaries of the information about to be provided as well as an opportunity for patients to repeat their understanding of the information[45].

Conclusion: a multi-tiered approach?

In this paper, we have tried to summarize many essential components of the informed consent process and provide insight into some of the causes of procedure-related anxiety and its management. Based on these findings, and on the authors' more than 130 years of combined procedure-related experience, we suggest development of a multi-tiered approach to the informed consent process that might include (i) a multimedia educational program that covers the informed consent process and acknowledges potential anxiety-provoking aspects of care, (ii) a short but concise preprocedure anxiety questionnaire that might help identify those individuals warranting medication or other anxiety-reducing interventions, and (iii) a universally acceptable written consent form that includes a technical description of the procedure along with a description of what the patient might actually *feel.*

Using this structured approach, the multimedia presentation could be translated into numerous languages and distributed using social media. This would increase the public's awareness of bronchoscopy, which, in turn, might help reduce procedure-related anxiety and enhance public trust. The questionnaire could be used to objectively identify those patients with procedure-related anxiety warranting additional emotional, psychological, or pharmacological support. The greater challenge is to develop a valid and universally acceptable written consent form, because so much of the information provided to patients must take into consideration a patient's goals, values, objectives, and cultural biases. A consent checklist, however, would assure documentation of the patient's knowledge and understanding of the procedure, the information being disclosed, the identity of the participants, the length of time devoted to the process, possible consequences of the patient's choice, and the physician's explicit opinion about the patient's decisional capacities. The likely outcome of any legal inquiry into the patient's competence could also be discussed, and family members or other care givers could be consulted in an attempt to identify what the patient's goals and wishes might have been, or whether certain interventions are, in fact, being performed with respect to the patient's best interests.

In the patient safety arena, the implementation of a structured review and checklist as part of a procedural pause (aka as "time out") performed immediately prior to open surgery or minimally invasive interventions has resulted in less physician and systems-based errors[46]. We propose that a similar process, implemented in a respectful, straight-forward, non-threatening manner that allows ample time for questions, would enhance the foundation of trust and shared decision-making so essential to the covenant that exists between physicians and their patients. Furthermore, this will likely reduce procedure-related anxiety and provide a legally binding and ethically unchallengeable process of true procedure-related informed consent.

References

1. Izard CE. The Psychology of Emotions. Plenum Press, New York, 1991 pg 287-308.
2. ACGME competency-based training reference, http://www.acgme.org/outcome/e-learn/e powerpoint.asp. Date access January 22, 2010.
3. Wahidi MM, Silvestri GA, Coakley RD, Ferguson JS, Shepherd RW, Moses L, Conforti J, Que L, Anstrom KJ, McGuire F, Colt HG, Downie GH. A prospective multi-center study of competency metrics and educational interventions in the learning of bronchoscopy among starting pulmonary fellows. *Chest*. 2010;137 (5):1040-1049.
4. Lechtzin N, Rugin HR, Jenckes M, White P, Zhou, Thompson DA, & Biette GB. Predictors of Pain Control in Patients Undergoing Flexible Bronchoscopy. *Am J Respir Crit Care Med.* 2000;162: 440-445.
5. Mehta AC. Don't Lose the Forest Through the Tree. *Am J Respir Crit Care Med.* 2002;166:1306-1307.
6. Colt HG, Prakash UBS, Offord KP. Bronchoscopy in North America: Survey by the American Association for Bronchology, 1999. *J Bronchol* 2000;7:8-25.
7. Desbiens NA, Wu AW, Broste SK, Wenger AF, Connors J, Lynn Y Lynn, Yasui Y, Phillips RS & Fulkerson W. Pain and Satisfaction with Pain Control in Seriously Ill Hospitalized Adults: Findings from The SUPPORT Research Investigation. *Crit. Care Med.* 1996;24(12):1953-1961.
8. Hicks JA, Jenkins JG. The Measurement of Pre-operative Anxiety. *J Royal Soc Med.*1988 91:517-519.
9. Speilberger CD, State-Trait Anxiety Inventory for Adults; *http://www. Mindgarden.com/products/staisad.htm*
10. Moerman N, Frits SAM, van Dam Muller, MJ Oosting H. The Amsterdam Pre-operative Anxiety and Information Scale (APAIS). *Anesth Analg.* 1996;82:445-451.
11. Boker A, Brownell L, Donen N; The Amsterdam Pre-operative Anxiety and Information Scale Provides a Simple and Reliable Measure of Pre-operative Anxiety. *Can J Anesth.* 2002;49:792-798.
12. Oldman M, Moore D, Collins S; Drug Patient Information Leaflets in Anaesthesia: Effect on Anxiety and Patient Satisfaction. *Br J Anaesth.* 2004;92:854-858.
13. Kijima Y, Hiroaki I, Fujita T, Mitono H; Relieving Anxiety by Entering the Operating Room on Foot. *Can J Anesth.* 2002;49:885-886.
14. Diette GB, Lechtzin N, Haponik E, Derotes A, Rubin HR; Distraction Therapy with Nature Sights and Sounds Reduces Pain During Flexible Bronchoscopy. *Chest.* 2003; 123:941-948.
15. Colt HG, Powers A, Shanks TG; Effect of Music on State Anxiety Scores in Patients Undergoing Fiberoptic Bronchoscopy. *Chest.* 1999;116:819-824.
16. Bampton P; Effect of Relaxation Music on Patient Tolerance of Gastrointestinal Endoscopic Procedures. *J Clin Gastroenterol.* 1997;25(1):343-346.
17. Want S, Kulkarni L, Doley J, Kain ZN; Music and Pre-operative Anxiety; A Randomized, Controlled Study. *Anesth Analg.* 2002;94:1489-1494.
18. Lee D, Henderson A, Shum D: The Effect of Music on Pre-procedure Anxiety in Hong Kong Chinese Day Patients. *J Clin Nursing.* 2004;13(3):297-303.
19. Lepage C, Drolet P, Girard M, Brenier Y, DeGagne R. Music Decreases Sedative Requirements during Spinal Anesthesia. *Anesth Analg.* 2001;93:912-916.
20. Tusek DL, DHurch JM, Strong SA, Grass JA, Fazio VW; Guided Imagery: A Significant Advance in the Care of Patients undergoing Elective Colorectal Surgery. *Dis Colon Rectum.* 1997;40:172-178.
21. Shaw C, Weaver CS, Schneider L; Conscious Sedation: A Multidisciplinary Team Approach. *J Post Anesth Nur.* 1996;11(1):13-19.
22. Hartsfield J, Clopton JR. Reducing Pre-Surgical Anxiety; A Possible Visitor Effect. *Soc Sci Med.* 1985;20(5):529-533.
23. Wells JK, Howard GS, Nowlin WF, Vargas MJ; Pre-Surgical Anxiety and Post-Surgical Pain and Adjustment: Effects of a Stress Inoculation Procedure. *J Consulting and Clin Psychol.* 1986;54(6):831-835.
24. Saadat H, Caldwel-Andrews A, Drummond-Lewis J, Zeev I; Effects of Hypnosis on Pre-Operative Anxiety in Adult Ambulatory Patients; *Anesthesiology.* 2005;103:A619.

25. Lechtzin N, Rugin HR, Jenckes M, White P, Zhou, Thompson DA, & Biette GB. Predictors of Pain Control in Patients Undergoing Flexible Bronchoscopy. *Am J Respir Crit Care Med.* 2000;162:440-445.
26. Code of Medical Ethics of the American Medical Association. Council of Ethics and Judicial Affairs. American Medical Society 2010-2011. Also see http://www.ama-assn.org/ama/pub/physician-resources/legal-topics/patient-physician-relationship-topics/informed-consent.page.
27. Bridson J, Hammond C, Leach A, Chester MR. Making consent patient centered. *BMJ.* 2003;327:1159-1161.
28. Berg JW, Appelbaum PJ. *Informed consent: legal theory and clinical practice.* 2nd ed. New York, Oxford University Press Inc. 2001.
29. Merz JF. An Empirical Analysis of the Medical Informed Consent Doctrine; Search for a "Standard of Disclosure *http//www.peircelaw.edu/vo2/winter/merz.htm;* pp 1-27.
30. Declaration of Helsinki. Downloaded from http://www.wma.net/e/policy/b3.htm. Accessed, November 20, 2008.
31. Colt HG and Mulnard RA. Writing an application for a human subjects institutional review board. *Chest.* 2006;130:1605-1607.
32. Bottrell MM, Fischback AH, Emanuel LL; Hospital Informed Consent Forms: Facilitating Quality patient-Physician Interaction. *Arch Surg.* 2000;135(1):23-26.
33. Beckman HB, Merkakis KM, Suchman AL, Frankel RM; The Doctor-Patient Relationship and Malpractice Lessons from Plaintiff Depositions. *Arch Intern Med.* 1994;154:1365-1370.
34. Claims RX: Clinical and Risk Management Perspectives; Informed Consent Update; The NORCAL Mutual Insurance Company Newsletter; March, 2007.
35. White-Bateman SR, Schumacher C, Sacco RL, Appelbaum PS; Consent for Intravenous Thrombolysis in Acute Stoke. *Arch Neurol.* 2007;64:785-792.
36. Agard A, Hermeren G, Herlitz J. Patient's Experiences of Intervention Trials on the Treatment of Myocardial Infarction: Is it Time to Adjust the Informed Consent Procedure to the Patient's Capacity? *Heart.* 2001;86:632-637.
37. Williams BF, French JK, White HD; Is Our Method of Obtaining Consent Appropriate for Randomised Controlled Trials in Acute Myocardial Infarction? *NZ Med J.* 1997;110:298-299.
38. Schmidt TA, Salo SD, Hughes JA, et al; SAEM Ethics Committee. Confronting the Ethical Challenges to Informed Consent in Emergency Medicine Research. *Acad Emerg Med.* 2004;11:1082-1089.
39. Akkad A, Jackson C, Dixon-Wood M, Taub N Habiba M; Informed Consent for Elective and Emergency Surgery; Questionnaire Study. *BJOG.* 2004;111:1133-1138.
40. Kondziolka DS, Pirris SM, Lunsford LD; Improving the Informed Consent Process for Surgery. *Neurosurgery.* 2006;58 (1):1184-1189.
41. Corbie-Smith G Thomas SB, M St. George DM. Distrust, race, and research. *J Gen Intem Med.* 1999;14:537-546.
42. Hattori H, Salzberg SM, Kiang WP,, Fujimiya T, Furuno J; The Patient's Right to Information in Japan—Legal Rules and Doctor's Opinions. *Soc Sci Med.* 1991;32(9): 1007-1016.
43. Ruhnke GW, Wilson SR, Akamatsu T, Takashima Y, Goldstein MK, Koenig BA, Hornberger JX, Raffin TA; Ethical Decision Making and Patient Autonomy: A Comparison of Physicians and Patients in Japan and the United States. *Chest.* 2000;118(4):1172-1182.
44. Quadrelli S, Colt HG, Lyons G, Cohen G. El respeto por la autonomia: cuanta informacion desean conocer los patientes para tomar decisiones (How much do patients want to know to make decisions?). *Medicina.* 2008;68 (3):198-204.
45. Dunn LB, Jeste DV; Enhancing Informed Consent for Research and Treatment. *Neuropsychopharmacology.* 2001;24:595-607.
46. Gawande Atul. *The Checklist Manifesto.* Metropolitan Books, Henry Holt and Company, New York, 2009.

Time Out (also referred to as Procedural Pause)*

Abstracted from Institute for Clinical Systems Improvement Guidelines: safe site invasive procedures non-operating room. Downloaded ICSI.org, February 1, 2010 from http://www.guideline.gov/summary/summary.aspx?ss=15&doc_id=13702

Active oral Time Out process

The Time Out is to be performed immediately prior to the start of the procedure and is the final safety stop before the procedure is begun. The purpose of the Time Out is to ensure that the correct patient, site, side, positioning and procedure to be performed are all correctly verified. In addition, it is an opportunity to validate that any related images, equipment or implants are available.

The Time Out is to be initiated by the provider and includes active verbal acknowledgment by all members of the team. The scalpel, needle or other cutting/incising device is not to be handed to the provider until the Time Out has been completed. While it is desirable to actively include the patient in the Time Out, it is not always possible, particularly if the patient is under the influence of sedating medications or is otherwise unable to participate.

It is recommended that a visual memory aid be used to trigger the initiation of the Time Out. For example, a "Time Out" sign or towel can be used to cover the scalpel, needle or cutting/incising device as a reminder to conduct the Time Out. When one of these aids is used, it is important to hand it off the sterile field at the conclusion of the Time Out so there is no potential for it to become retained in the patient.

Every Time Out must include the following standard elements:

- Patient identity, using a minimum of two identifiers
- Procedure(s) to be performed (including internal and/or external laterality, multiples and/or level)
- Patient positioning if not already verified
- Procedure side, site and/or level including visualization of the provider's initials if applicable
- As appropriate, imaging, equipment, implants or special requirements (e.g., pre-procedure antibiotic administration)

The provider may delegate the Time Out elements to the nurse or other member of the team, but the initiation of the Time Out should be the responsibility of the provider. The nurse or other team member may refer to the patient consent for the Time Out elements. However, prior to its use, the consent must have been validated against other documents, such as history and physical, radiology or pathology reports, progress notes, etc.

During the Time Out, each person in the procedure room must stop what he or she is doing and actively participate in the process. Involved staff may include the provider, resident, student, anesthesia, scrub, nurse and/or vendors whenever present. No individual is exempt from the process. Active participation requires each individual to state clearly and loudly that they agree with the elements of the Time Out. The scalpel, needle or other cutting/incising device is not to be handed to the provider until the Time Out has been completed. If a member of the team refuses to actively participate in the Time Out, the scalpel, needle or cutting/incising device is not handed to the provider until that individual is replaced and the Time Out completed.

Environmental distractions are to be eliminated as much as possible during the Time Out. For example, music is turned off, pagers are set on vibrate, talking other than participation in Time Out ceases and no staff are permitted to enter or exit the room. If during the Time Out an interruption or distraction occurs (pager goes off or an individual enters the room), the Time Out must be restarted.

Additional Time Outs are to be performed when there are two or more different procedures performed on the same patient during the same procedure period, whether or not the procedures involve a new procedure team. The process and elements of the Time Out as described above must occur prior to the start of the next procedure.

If the patient needs to be repositioned during the procedure and this repositioning affects the patient's presentation (i.e., the patient is turned prone), an abbreviated Time Out including the site, side, level and/or visualization of the provider's initials will be conducted. The Time Out process will be the same as described above (e.g., elimination of distractions, active participation).

Universal Precautions

Excerpt from the Fact Sheet Center for Disease Control:
Provided for informational and educational use only
Downloaded February 1, 2010, from
http://www.cdc.gov/ncidod/dhqp/bp_universal_precautions.html#

"Universal precautions," as defined by CDC, are a set of precautions designed to prevent transmission of human immunodeficiency virus (HIV), hepatitis B virus (HBV), and other bloodborne pathogens when providing first aid or health care. Under universal precautions, blood and certain body fluids of all patients are considered potentially infectious for HIV, HBV and other bloodborne pathogens.

Universal precautions took the place of and eliminated the need for the isolation category "Blood and Body Fluid Precautions" in the 1983 CDC Guidelines for Isolation Precautions in Hospitals. However, implementing universal precautions does not eliminate the need for other isolation precautions, such as droplet precautions for influenza, airborne isolation for pulmonary tuberculosis, or contact isolation for methicillin-resistant *Staphylococcus aureus*.

Universal precautions apply to blood, other body fluids containing visible blood, semen, and vaginal secretions. Universal precautions also apply to tissues and to the following fluids: cerebrospinal, synovial, pleural, peritoneal, pericardial, and amniotic fluids. Universal precautions do not apply to feces, nasal secretions, sputum, sweat, tears, urine, and vomitus unless they contain visible blood. Universal precautions do not apply to saliva except when visibly contaminated with blood or in the dental setting where blood contamination of saliva is predictable.

Universal precautions involve the use of protective barriers such as gloves, gowns, aprons, masks, or protective eyewear, which can reduce the risk of exposure of the health care worker's skin or mucous membranes to potentially infective materials. In addition, under universal precautions, it is recommended that all health care workers take precautions to prevent injuries caused by needles, scalpels, and other sharp instruments or devices.

Pregnant health care workers are not known to be at greater risk of contracting HIV infection than are health care workers who are not pregnant; however, if a health care worker develops HIV infection during pregnancy, the infant is at risk of infection resulting from perinatal transmission. Because of this risk, pregnant health care workers should be especially familiar with, and strictly adhere to, precautions to minimize the risk of HIV transmission.

GLOVING, GOWNING, MASKING, AND OTHER PROTECTIVE BARRIERS

All health care workers should routinely use appropriate barrier precautions to prevent skin and mucous membrane exposure during contact with any patient's blood or body fluids that require universal precautions.

Recommendations for the use of gloves are presented in detail in the Morbidity and Mortality Weekly Report dated June 24, 1988, which is available by calling the National AIDS Information Hotline at 1-800-342-2437 or the National AIDS Information Clearinghouse at 1-800-458-5231.

Gloves should be worn:

- for touching blood and body fluids requiring universal precautions, mucous membranes, or non-intact skin of all patients, and
- for handling items or surfaces soiled with blood or body fluids to which universal precautions apply.

Gloves should be changed after contact with each patient. Hands and other skin surfaces should be washed immediately or as soon as patient safety permits if contaminated with blood or body fluids requiring universal precautions. Hands should be washed immediately after gloves are removed. Gloves should reduce the incidence of blood contamination of hands during phlebotomy, but they cannot prevent penetrating injuries caused by needles or other sharp instruments. Institutions that judge routine gloving for all phlebotomies is not necessary should periodically reevaluate their policy. Gloves should always be available to health care workers who wish to use them for phlebotomy. In addition, the following general guidelines apply:

1. Use gloves for performing phlebotomy when the health care worker has cuts, scratches, or other breaks in his/her skin.
2. Use gloves in situations where the health care worker judges that hand contamination with blood may occur, e.g., when performing phlebotomy on an uncooperative patient.
3. Use gloves for performing finger and/or heel sticks on infants and children.
4. Use gloves when persons are receiving training in phlebotomy.

Masks and protective eyewear or face shields should be worn by health care workers to prevent exposure of mucous membranes of the mouth, nose, and eyes during procedures that are likely to generate droplets of blood or body fluids requiring universal precautions. Gowns or aprons should be worn during procedures that are likely to generate splashes of blood or body fluids requiring universal precautions.

All health care workers should take precautions to prevent injuries caused by needles, scalpels, and other sharp instruments or devices during procedures; when cleaning used instruments; during disposal of used needles; and when handling sharp instruments after procedures. To prevent needlestick injuries, needles should not be recapped by hand, purposely bent or broken by hand, removed from disposable syringes, or otherwise manipulated by hand. After they are used, disposable syringes and needles, scalpel blades, and other sharp items should be placed in puncture-resistant containers for disposal. The puncture-resistant containers should be located as close as practical to the use area. All reusable needles should be placed in a puncture-resistant container for transport to the reprocessing area.

General infection control practices should further minimize the already minute risk for salivary transmission of HIV. These infection control practices include the use of gloves for digital examination of mucous membranes and endotracheal suctioning, handwashing after exposure to saliva, and minimizing the need for emergency mouth-to-mouth resuscitation by making mouthpieces and other ventilation devices available for use in areas where the need for resuscitation is predictable.

SECTION 6

Practical Approach Sessions

Interactive Patient-centered
Practical Approach to Procedural Decision-making exercises

USER INSTRUCTIONS

Practical Approach Workshops

The purpose of these practical approach sessions is to help learners think through the decision making process. Often, instructors will use a practical approach to help students gain insights into the strategy and planning, technical performance, and response to complications elements of a minimally invasive procedure.

These exercises are done orally, and the assessment is subjective, based on the instructor's perception of how the learner responds to questions and outlines a procedural strategy. Learners are taught to use scientific evidence as well as expert opinion to formulate plans and achieve desired results. A dialogue is thus engendered between instructor and student in order to address alternatives and differences in technique, as well as expected outcomes.

It is expected that sessions last no more than 30 minutes. The learner may be given a scenario, and using a model of the four box approach the learner might be asked to address each of the four boxes, with specific emphasis on one or two items based on instructor preference. Numerous exercises are available on the Bronchoscopy.org website, but any scenario the instructor creates can be used for teaching purposes.

Four Box Approach

Initial Evaluation	Procedural Strategies and planning
1. Physical examination, complementary tests, and functional status assessment 2. Patient's significant comorbidities 3. Patient's support system (also includes family) 4. Patient preferences and expectations (also includes family)	1. Indications, contraindications, and expected results 2. Operator and team experience and expertise 3. Risk-benefits analysis and therapeutic alternatives 4. Respect for persons (Informed Consent and ethics issues)
Procedural Techniques and results	**Long term Management Plan**
1. Anesthesia and other perioperative care 2. Techniques and instrumentation 3. Anatomic dangers and other risks 4. Results and procedure-related complications	1. Outcome assessment 2. Follow-up tests, visits, and procedures 3. Referrals to medical, surgical, or palliative/end of life subspecialty care 4. Quality improvement and team evaluation of clinical encounter

The Patient-centered practical approach is an interactive learning program:

- The purpose of *The Practical Approach* is to help learners gain the cognitive, technical, experiential, and affective skills necessary to perform bronchoscopy. Competency is sought in the three major elements of a procedure; strategy and planning, execution, and response to procedure-related adverse events or complications.
- Using a four box approach inspired from Albert Jonsen's[1] classic work in medical ethics, learners rationalize various components of the decision making process.
    - By working through case scenarios, learners are prompted to think about the how and why of their actions, based on background information, pertinent literature, and experience.
    - Consistent with the ACGME professionalism competency guides[2,3], case scenarios prompt learners to address various components of the informed consent process, and discuss outcomes based on possible as well as real results.
- *The Practical Approach* helps learners become competent bronchoscopists according to current recommendations set forth by the American College of Graduate Medical Education[4] whereby trainees learn to:
    - Gather essential and accurate information about their patients.
    - Make informed decisions about diagnostic and therapeutic interventions based on patient information and preferences, up-to-date scientific evidence and clinical judgment.
    - Use information technology to support patient care decisions and patient education.
    - Develop patient management plans.
    - Counsel and educate patients and their families.
    - Communicate effectively and demonstrate caring and respectful behaviors when interacting with patients and their families.
    - Provide healthcare services aimed at preventing health problems or maintaining health.
    - Work with healthcare professionals, including those from other disciplines to provide patient-focused care.

References

1. Jonsen AR, Siegler M, Winslade WJ. Clinical Ethics. 6th Ed, McGraw Hill, NY 2006.
2. ACGME Web site:http//www.acgme.org/outcome/comp/compfull.asp
3. Apelgren K. ACGME e-Bulletin. August 2006
4. ACGME Competencies at http://www.acgme.org
5. *Patient-centered approach to central airways disorders.* Colt HG and Murgu S, Published, Elsevier Press 2012.

Practical Approach Module

Scenario: Flexible bronchoscopy with BAL in a deaf patient with suspected pulmonary lymphangitic carcinomatosis [Abstracted from www.Bronchoscopy.org]

Based on the information presented below, please describe your procedural decision making using The Practical Approach to Procedural Decision making. Do your best to complete each item of the Four Boxes. If the case scenario contains no information pertaining to an item, please address it as NOT AVAILABLE. Note that each case scenario may have greater emphasis on one or more items listed in the "Practical Approach".

MM is a 72 year old man with stage IV adenocarcinoma of the lung admitted for progressive dyspnea. He has undergone multiple chemotherapy regimens. Four months before admission he was started on tyrosine kinase inhibitors. He has increasing shortness of breath, fatigue, dry cough, and weight loss for several weeks. He also has COPD with FEV1 35% predicted. The patient is deaf and lives with his 33 year old son. The patient's Karnofsky status is 50.

Chest radiograph shows diffuse bilateral interstitial infiltrates and an ill-defined opacity at the right lung base. Computed tomography scan reveals intralobular septal thickening and consolidation in the right middle lobe which was the site of the primary tumor.

Physical examination reveals a temperature of 37.6 blood pressure 112/74 pulse 92 respiratory rate 22 and SaO2 91% on Room Air. He is in no acute distress but is ill-appearing and cachectic. His examination is normal except for diffuse bilateral crackles with decreased breath sounds at the right base and evidence of digital clubbing.

Laboratory findings reveal: Sodium 136; BUN 33; Creatinine 1.7; Glucose 124; CBC showing WBC 12.3, Neutrophil 78% with no bands, Hemoglobin 13.3, and Platelets 163,000. Blood cultures are negative; urinalysis is negative; sputum gram stain is negative (cultures are pending).

The oncology team has formulated a differential diagnosis that includes lymphangitic carcinomatosis, pulmonary infection, and drug-related pneumonitis. This has prompted consultation and a request for flexible bronchoscopy.

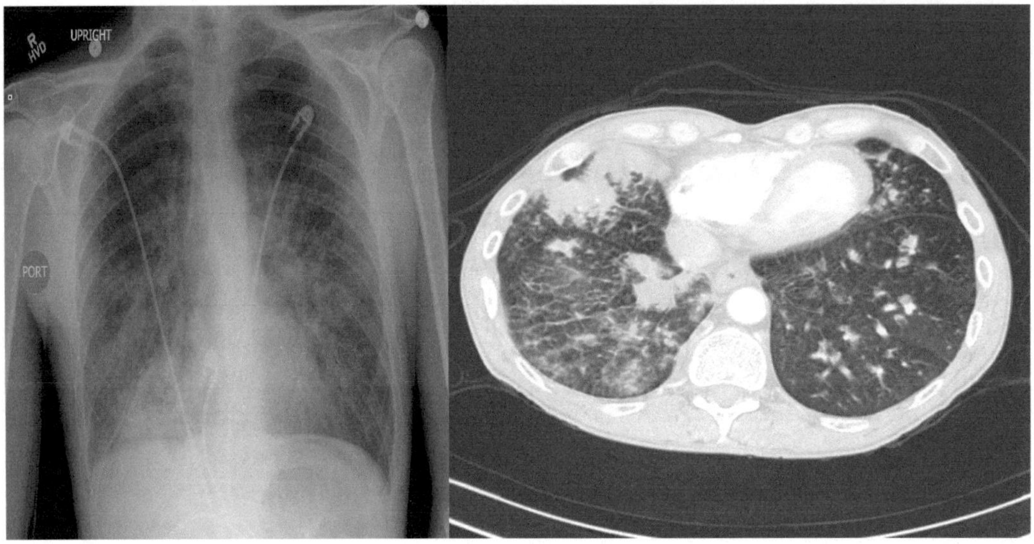

After addressing items of the four boxes:

- Describe radiographic characteristics of pulmonary lymphangitic carcinomatosis.
- Define the role of bronchioloalveolar lavage and transbronchial lung biopsy in the diagnosis of lymphangitic spread.
- Should transbronchial lung biopsy be performed in this patient?

Initial Evaluation	Procedural Strategies
1. Physical examination, complementary tests, and functional status assessment 2. Patient's significant co-morbidities 3. patient's support system (also includes family) 4. Patient preferences and expectations (also includes family)	1. Indications, contraindications, and expected results 2. Operator and team experience and expertise 3. Risk-benefits analysis and therapeutic alternatives 4. Respect for persons (Informed Consent)
Procedural Techniques and results	**Long term Management Plan**
1. Anesthesia and other perioperative care 2. Techniques and instrumentation 3. Anatomic dangers and other risks 4. Results and procedure-related complications	1. Outcome assessment 2. Follow-up tests, visits, and procedures 3. Referrals to medical, surgical, or palliative/end of life subspecialty care 4. Quality improvement and team evaluation of clinical encounter

Practical Approach bandw

Bronchoscopy for suspected pulmonary lymphangitic carcinomatosis

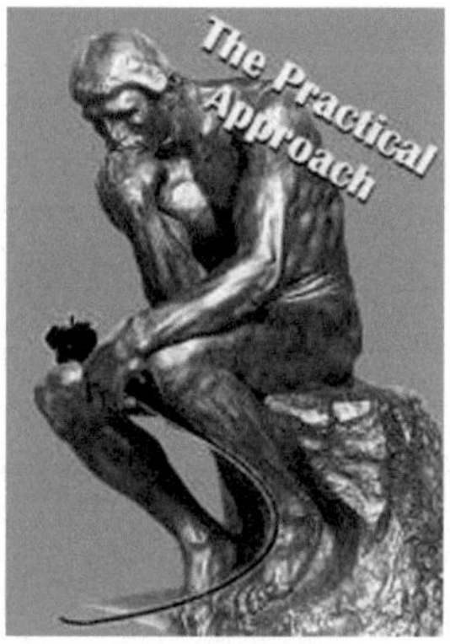

- Learning Objectives
  - To identify radiographic characteristics of pulmonary lymphangitic carcinomatosis.
  - To define the role of bronchioloalveolar lavage and transbronchial lung biopsy for diagnosis of lymphangitic spread.
  - To identify ways of obtaining informed consent from a deaf person.

Bronchoscopy International

Case description

- G.G. is a 72 year old man with stage IV adenocarcinoma of the lung admitted for progressive dyspnea. He has undergone multiple chemotherapy regimens. Four months before admission he was started on tyrosine kinase inhibitors.
- He has increasing shortness of breath, fatigue, dry cough, and weight loss for several weeks. The patient has COPD with FEV1 35% predicted and is deaf.
- He lives with his 33 year old son. Karnoksky status is 50.
- Chest radiograph shows diffuse bilateral interstitial infiltrates and an ill-defined opacity at the right lung base.
- Computed tomography scan reveals intralobular septal thickening and consolidation in the right middle lobe which was the site of the primary tumor.
- The oncology team has formulated a differential diagnosis that includes lymphangitic carcinomatosis, pulmonary infection, and drug-related pneumonitis. Pulmonary consultation is requested for bronchoscopy.

Bronchoscopy International

The Practical Approach

Initial Evaluation	Procedural Strategies
• Examination & functional status • Significant comorbidities • Support system • Patient preferences & expectations	• Indications, contraindications, & results • Team experience • Risk-benefits analysis & therapeutic alternatives • Informed Consent
Techniques and Results	**Long term Management**
• Anesthesia & peri-operative care • Techniques & instrumentation • Anatomic dangers & other risks • Results & procedure-related complications	• Outcome assessment • Follow-up tests & procedures • Referrals • Quality improvement

Bronchoscopy International

Initial Evaluation

- Physical Exam
  - T 37.6 BP 112/74 P 92 R 22 SaO_2 91% RA
  - General: NAD but ill-appearing, A&Ox4, cachectic
  - HEENT: PERRLA, sclera anicteric, no neck LAD
  - Chest: diffuse bilateral crackles with decreased BS at right lung base, no wheezing
  - Heart: RRNR S_1 S_2 no murmur
  - Abd: soft, NT, ND, normoactive BS
  - Ext: +digital clubbing, no edema or cyanosis
- Labs
  - Chem panel: Na+ 136 BUN 33 Crt 1.7 Glu 124
  - CBC: WBC 12.3 Neutrophil 78% no bands Hgb 13.3 Plt 163
  - Blood cx NGTD, U/A neg, sputum cx pending (Gram stain neg)

Bronchoscopy International

Initial Evaluation

- Left: chest radiograph shows diffuse bilateral interstitial infiltrates and an ill- defined opacity at the right lung base. Right: computed tomography scan reveals intralobular septal thickening and consolidation in the right middle lobe which was the site of the primary tumor.

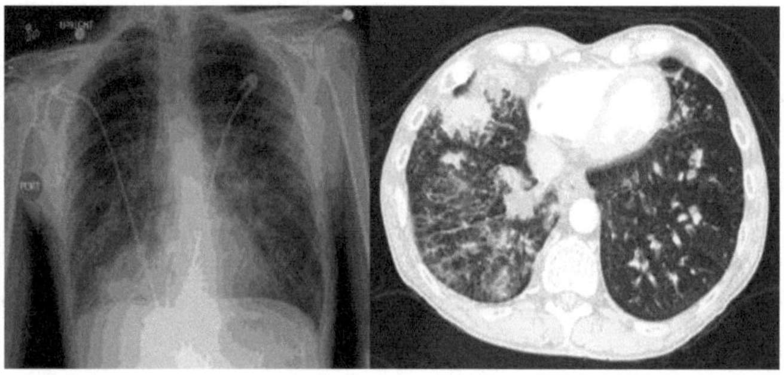

Bronchoscopy International

Initial Evaluation

- Functional status assessment
  - Karnofsky status score 50
- Significant co-morbidities
  - Advanced COPD, HTN, chronic renal insufficiency, poor functional capacity
- Support system
  - Lives with wife, has 3 children who are supportive
- Preferences and expectations
  - Realistic and understands severity of disease

Bronchoscopy International

Karnofsky Performance Status Scale Definitions Rating (%) Criteria

- Able to carry on normal activity and to work; no special care needed
  - 100: normal; no complaints; no evidence of disease
  - 90: able to carry on normal activity; minor signs or symptoms of disease
  - 80: normal activity with effort; some signs or symptoms of disease
- Unable to work; able to live at home and care for most personal needs; varying amount of assistance needed
  - 70: cares for self; unable to carry on normal activity or to do active work
  - 60: requires occasional assistance, but is able to care for most of his personal needs
  - **50: requires considerable assistance and frequent medical care**
- Unable to care for self; requires equivalent of institutional or hospital care; disease may be progressing rapidly
  - 40: disabled; requires special care and assistance
  - 30: severely disabled; hospital admission is indicated although death not imminent
  - 20: very sick; hospital admission necessary; active supportive treatment necessary
  - 10: moribund; fatal processes progressing rapidly
  - 0: deceased

Bronchoscopy International

Procedural Strategies

- Indications for bronchoscopy
  - Diagnosis of lymphangitic carcinomatosis
  - Evaluation of presence of infection
    - ♦ Bacterial vs. fungal vs. viral
- Contraindications for bronchoscopy
  - No history of recent MI or arrhythmia
  - History of advanced COPD
    - ♦ 5% of COPD patients with bronchoscopy-related complication compared to 0.6% in patients with normal lung function
    - ♦ Especially at risk:
      - FEV_1/FVC <50% or
      - FEV_1 <1L and FEV_1/FVC <69%
    - ♦ Consider pre-procedure spirometry in severe COPD (increased concern if FEV_1 <40%)
    - ♦ Use sedation and O_2 carefully in patients with elevated CO_2 (concern for retention)

Bronchoscopy International

Procedural Strategies

- Operator and team experience
- Risks of bronchoscopy
    - Mortality rate: 0.01-0.04%
    - Complication rate: 0.12-0.30%
  - Oversedation
    - ♦ May cause desaturations or CO_2 retention
  - Bronchospasm
    - ♦ Premedicate with bronchodilator to reduce decrease in FEV_1
      – Data in asthmatic patients
  - Laryngospasm
  - Hypoxemia
    - ♦ Maintain SaO_2 > 90% in perioperative setting
  - Bleeding
    - ♦ UCI policy is to check preoperative CBC and coagulation panel
    - ♦ BTS recommends routine preop coags before bronchoscopy

Bronchoscopy International

Procedural Strategies

- Informed consent for the hearing-impaired
- When deaf patients sign consent forms, they often do so without understanding them
    - ♦ Many believe forms are malpractice waivers
  - Involvement of an interpreter is indispensable
  - Allows physician to
    - ♦ Obtain thorough history and proper examination
    - ♦ Ensure that patient understands risks and benefits of procedure
    - ♦ Establish effective communication and environment of caring and trust
  - Communicate through writing when possible as opposed to lip-reading

Bronchoscopy International

Procedural Techniques and Results

- Anesthesia: moderate sedation
  - Midazolam
    - Well tolerated
    - Less than 10% exhibit prolonged effect from impaired metabolism
    - Initial dose of 2 mg followed after 2 minutes by increments of 1 mg/min if needed
  - Propofol: monitor for hypotension
  - Flumazenil: benzodiazepine antagonist
    - Short elimination time allows re-sedation
    - Usual initial dosage: 250-500 micrograms
- Perioperative care
  - Continuous oxygen with monitoring
  - Preoperative bronchodilator
  - Viscous and liquid Lidocaine
- Procedure-related complications

*reference

Bronchoscopy International

Long-term Management Plan

- BAL was performed and revealed malignant cells consistent with adenocarcinoma
- Diagnosis of lymphangitic carcinomatosis was discussed with patient and given poor prognosis a palliative care consult was considered
- Patient was discharged home with hospice
  - Patient and family expressed satisfaction with care and management by all subspecialty and ancillary teams

Bronchoscopy International

Q 1: What are the specific CT characteristics of pulmonary lymphangitic carcinomatosis and how do they differ from those of tyrosine kinase inhibitor-induced interstitial pneumonitis?

- HRCT findings in lymphangitic carcinomatosis
  - Irregular, nodular, and/or smooth interlobular septal thickening
  - Thickening of fissures as result of involvement of lymphatics concentrated in subpleural interstitium
  - Preservation of normal parenchymal architecture at level of second pulmonary lobule
  - Peribronchovascular thickening
  - Centrilobular peribronchovascular thickening predominating over interlobular septal thickening in a minority of patients
  - Polygonal arcades or polygons with prominence of centrilobular bronchovascular bundle in association with interlobular septal thickening (50%)
  - Mediastinal and/or hilar lymphadenopathy (30-50%)
  - Pleural effusions (30-50%)
- Findings can be unilateral or bilateral and focal or diffuse

Bronchoscopy International

Q 1: What are the specific CT characteristics of pulmonary lymphangitic carcinomatosis and how do they differ from those of tyrosine kinase inhibitor-induced interstitial pneumonitis?

- HRCT findings in tyrosine kinase-induced interstitial pneumonitis
  - Diffuse interstitial markings and increased radiodensities
  - **Ground glass opacities**
  - Multiple centrilobular nodules
  - Focal air trapping
  - Pleural effusion
  - **Extensive fibrosis and honeycombing with traction bronchiectasis in chronic and advanced disease**

Bronchoscopy International

Lymphangitic carcinomatosis

Smooth and nodular interlobular septal thickening (black arrow)

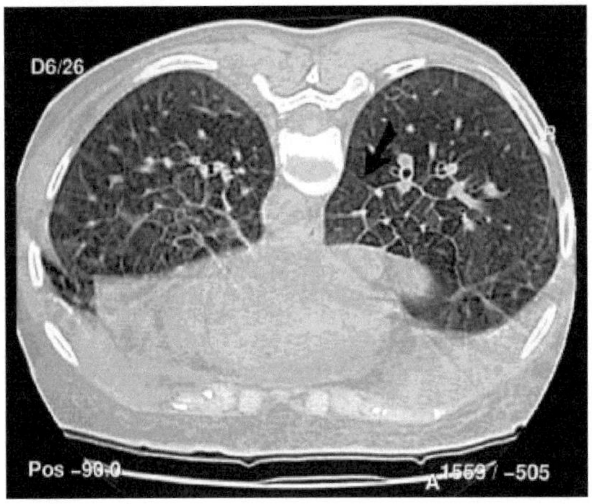

Bronchoscopy International

Lymphangitic carcinomatosis

Prominent axial interstitium with thickened bronchovascular bundles (solid arrow). Also thickening of fissure secondary to involvement of subpleural lymphatics (open arrow).

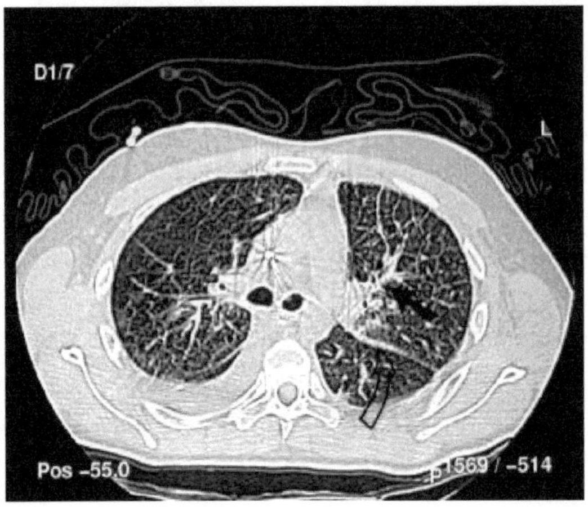

Bronchoscopy International

Tyrosine kinase-induced interstitial pneumonitis

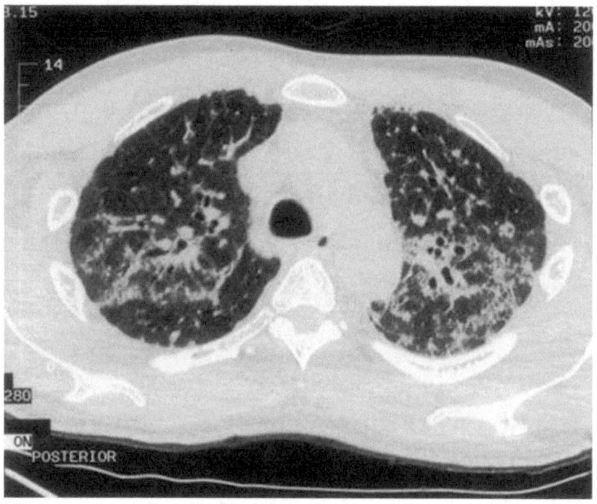

Bronchoscopy International

Q 2: What is the expected yield of bronchoalveolar lavage for diagnosing lymphangitic carcinomatosis, and how does this yield compare with that of transbronchial lung biopsy?

- Transbronchial lung biopsy
  - Goal is to replace more invasive open lung or transthoracic needle biopsy
  - 19 patients with diffuse interstitial disease underwent flexible bronchoscopy with transbronchial biopsy
    - ♦ Lymphangitic carcinomatosis was established in 6 (32%) of patients
      - One patient developed 30% pneumothorax which was treated with chest tube evacuation
  - The diffuse bronchial and peribronchial lymphatic involvement demonstrated suggests that TBLB should be the procedure of choice in diagnosis of lymphangitic carcinomatosis
  - Aranda C et al. Transbronchial lung biopsy in the diagnosis of lymphangitic carcinomatosis. Cancer 1978;42:1995-8.

Bronchoscopy International

Q 2: What is the expected yield of bronchoalveolar lavage for diagnosing lymphangitic carcinomatosis, and how does this yield compare with that of transbronchial lung biopsy?

- Bronchoalveolar lavage
  - Retrospective analysis, 12 patients with known neoplastic disease and diffuse pulmonary infiltrates consistent with lymphangitic carcinomatosis
    - ♦ BAL correctly identified 5/5 (100%)
      - No complications
    - ♦ Bronchial washing 4/7 (57%)
    - ♦ Bronchial brushing 2/5 (40%)
    - ♦ Transbronchial lung biopsy 4/9 (44%)
  - One patient with significant pulmonary hemorrhage
  - Conclusion: BAL should be performed to confirm diagnosis before proceeding to biopsy, especially when risks of pneumothorax and hemorrhage are excessive
  - The value of bronchial washings and bronchoalveolar lavage in the diagnosis of lymphangitic carcinomatosis. Chest 1998;94:1028-30

Bronchoscopy International

Q 3: Should you perform transbronchial lung biopsy in this case? If so, why? If not, why not?

- History of advanced COPD with increased concern for pneumothorax
- History of chronic renal insufficiency with concern for platelet dysfunction and increased risk of bleeding
- Evidence showing BAL as the initial test of choice in diagnosis of lymphangitic carcinomatosis
  - Consider TBLB if BAL is non-diagnostic and patient wishes to pursue further diagnosis and treatment

Prepared with the assistance of Paul Huang M.D.

www.bronchoscopy.org
Bronchoscopy International

SECTION 7

Proctored Bronchoscopy

Proctored patient-care in the procedural setting

The learner is observed performing one or more flexible bronchoscopies in a real patient setting. Checklists and bronchoscopy assessment tools are used to document performance.

USER INSTRUCTIONS

Proctored Flexible Bronchoscopy

The purpose of proctoring a procedure is to document that the learner is indeed able to perform all the elements of flexible bronchoscopy independently. These include strategy and planning, technique, patient safety measures and the ability to respond appropriately to procedure-related adverse events.

A ten-point checklist can be used for grading purposes. If warranted, the bronchoscopy assessment tools can also be used. The overall assessment must also include the faculty's general observations of the learner's practices during the course of training. From an assessment perspective, this is the last item with which to "score" a learner's ability to competently perform bronchoscopy. The intensity with which proctoring occurs, and the number of "proctored" cases that may be required within a training program are left to each program director's discretion.

PROCTORED FLEXIBLE BRONCHOSCOPY 10-Point CHECKLIST*

Learner ______________________ **Training Year** ______________

Faculty ______________________ **Date** ______________

☐ **Simulation Bronchoscopy Workshop** ☐ **Patient-based Bronchoscopy Scenario**

Educational Item* Items 1-10 are scored 10 points each (no partial points given)	**Satisfactory Yes/No**
1. Formulation of effective plan and strategy: ☐ Informed consent obtained, signed and in medical record ☐ History and physical ☐ Review imaging studies ☐ Cost-effective practice ☐ Use of information resources ☐ Applies evidence-based medicine ☐ Use of systems resources	Yes / No
2. Patient safety: ☐ ASA assessment ☐ Airway assessment ☐ Allergies ☐ Medications ☐ Comorbidities	Yes / No
3. Patient safety: ☐ Positioning ☐ Supplemental oxygen ☐ Vital signs ☐ Suction ☐ Bite-block and/or ET tube if applicable ☐ Verifies ability to respond to complications and accessibility of resuscitation equipment	Yes / No
4. Patient and procedural team safety: ☐ Protection from radiation/lead shielding; badge use ☐ Eye protection ☐ Knowledgeable use of fluoroscopy ☐ Hand disinfection ☐ Universal precautions ☐ "Time-Out".	Yes / No
5. Procedure: ☐ Premedication ☐ Moderate sedation ☐ Topical anesthetic	Yes / No
6. Procedure: ☐ Scope insertion ☐ Topical anesthetic ☐ Passage through vocal cords ☐ Empathy and communication with patient	Yes / No
7. Procedure: ☐ Inspection of tracheobronchial tree ☐ Identification of abnormalities ☐ Atraumatic removal of bronchoscope	Yes / No
8. Procedure: ☐ BAL ☐ Mucosal biopsy ☐ Lung biopsy ☐ Brush ☐ TBNA ☐ EBUS	Yes / No
9. Communication with staff, patient, and patient family ☐ Puts needs of patient first ☐ Punctuality ☐ Respect ☐ Listening skills ☐ Personal appearance ☐ Initiative & Motivation ☐ Empathy ☐ Honesty ☐ Accepts responsibility	Yes / No
10. Documentation/procedure note ☐ Informative ☐ Accurate ☐ Communication with colleagues	Yes / No

* Each of the 10 items contains all of the elements required by ACGME (patient care, medical knowledge, practice-based learning and improvement, interpersonal communication skills, professionalism, and systems-based practice).

FINAL GRADE PASS FAIL **SCORE** ______/100

USER INSTRUCTIONS

Proctored Flexible Bronchoscopy Checklist

Educational Item*   Items 1-10 each scored 10 points (no partial points given)
1. Formulation of effective plan and strategy   ☐ Informed consent obtained, signed and in medical record ☐ History and physical ☐ Review imaging studies   ☐ Cost-effective practice ☐ Use of information resources ☐ Applies evidence-based medicine   ☐ Use of systems resources   * The instructor should be certain that the student has obtained the informed consent and that it is signed and in the chart. The student should be able to describe pertinent clinical and radiographic findings and to use evidence-based medicine in addition to any other information gained from other resources, such as faculty expert opinion, advice, and requests by referring physicians, to justify the procedure being performed. The student should be able to describe the use of institutional resources, and use them according to institutional practices, such as fluoroscopy, ultrasound, computed tomography, electrocautery and other instruments and equipment. This also includes nursing surveillance, respiratory therapy assistance, need for procedure suite, operating theater or intensive care unit. Cost-effectiveness can be discussed in regards to other diagnostic or therapeutic modalities, but also how bronchoscopy may or may not increase or decrease health-related expenditures in the context of the patient's diagnosis and treatment plan.
2. Patient safety: ☐ ASA assessment ☐ Airway assessment ☐ Allergies ☐ Medications ☐ Comorbidities   * ASA and Airway assessments should be performed according to the institution's guidelines. Allergies, medications, especially anticoagulants and antiplatelet agents should be noted, comorbidities that might increase the risk of adverse events should also be described and identified.
3. Patient safety: ☐ Positioning ☐ Supplemental oxygen ☐ Vital signs ☐ Suction ☐ Bite-block and/or ET tube if applicable   ☐ Verifies ability to respond to complications and accessibility of resuscitation equipment   *These measures should be taken according to institutional biases and protocols.
4. Patient and procedural team safety: ☐ Protection from radiation/lead shielding, badge use ☐ Eye protection ☐ Knowledgeable use of fluoroscopy   ☐ Hand disinfection ☐ Universal precautions ☐ "Time-Out".   *Students should be observed as they comply with these safety measures. Additional information pertaining to time-out, universal precautions, and knowledge of fluoroscopy are provided in the modules. Protocols may vary among institutions.
5. Procedure: ☐ Premedication ☐ Moderate sedation ☐ Topical anesthetic   *These should be administered according to institutional biases and according to protocols.

6. Procedure:
☐ Scope insertion ☐ Topical anesthetic ☐ Passage through vocal cords
☐ Empathy and communication with patient

*Done according to institutional practices. Empathy and communication with the patient should be observed. Students should be able to speak comfortably and reassuringly with their patient. Open dialogues should be encouraged to enhance confidence and decrease patient anxiety.

7. Procedure:
☐ Inspection of tracheobronchial tree ☐ Identification of abnormalities ☐ Atraumatic removal of bronchoscope

*Performed according to institutional practices.

8. Procedure:
☐ BAL ☐ Mucosal biopsy ☐ Lung biopsy ☐ Brush ☐ TBNA ☐ EBUS

*Performed according to institutional practices. It is recognized that not all patients will undergo all of these procedures, therefore, if the institution desires, a different proctored checklist can be completed for each (or each set) of the procedures listed.

9. Communication with staff, patient, and patient family
☐ Puts needs of patient first ☐ Punctuality ☐ Respect ☐ Listening skills ☐ Personal appearance
☐ Initiative & Motivation ☐ Empathy ☐ Honesty ☐ Accepts responsibility

*These are for the most part subjective assessments, and also require feedback from nursing staff. Students should be told that they will be judged on these items during the course of their training, so that they can obtain feedback from their instructors and improve their performance in these areas.

10. **Documentation/procedure note**
☐ Informative ☐ Accurate ☐ Communication with colleagues

*Procedure notes may vary according to institution; however, in general, the note should be informative, telling a story about the procedure that referring physicians can understand. The note should be accurate regarding what was done, why it was done, and how it was done. Procedure-related adverse events should be described. Communication with colleagues should be observed, by watching how the student interacts with the nursing team, other physicians, and with referring physicians. While this element is also, for the most part subjective, in general, communication should be informative, accurate polite, and considerate.

* Each of the 10 items contains all of the elements required by ACGME (patient care, medical knowledge, practice-based learning and improvement, interpersonal communication skills, professionalism, and systems-based practice).

FINAL GRADE PASS FAIL **SCORE** _______/100

SECTION 8

Bronchoscopy Assessment Tools And User Instructions*

- BSTAT (Bronchoscopy Skills and Tasks)
- BSTAT-TBLB/TBNA
- BSAT (Bronchoscopy Self-Assessment Tool)
- BSTAT, BSTAT-TBLB/TBNA and BSAT User instructions
- Questions and answers for modules 1-6 of the

Essential Flexible Bronchoscopist©

**All assessment tools, including BSTAT quiz and BSTAT-TBLB/TBNA quiz and all post-tests for the Essential Flexible Bronchoscopist© are available in a separate appendix.*

Scoring Recommendations for Bronchoscopy Assessment Tools

(BSTAT, BSTAT-TBLB/TBNA, BSAT)

The goal of these assessment tools is to be able to monitor a learner's progress along the learning curve from *novice* (Score < 60) to *advanced beginner* (Score 60-79), *intermediate* (score 80-99), and *competent* (score 100). The instructor should be able to ascertain, by observing the learner's performance (For BSTAT tools, this could be done on a once or twice a year basis) that each of the ten elements in each tool are covered satisfactorily. Repeated testing will demonstrate increases in knowledge and technical skill acquisition as the student climbs the learning curve from novice to advanced beginner, intermediate and competent bronchoscopist for the procedure being assessed.

To maximize objective scoring, each task has been defined explicitly in this user manual for each checklist and assessment tool. Participation in specially-designed Train-the-Trainers courses is encouraged to assist with standardization and to help instructors use this program to its fullest potential.

Scores can be plotted on a graph, and each institution or training program can choose its own cut-offs for a PASS grade, although we recommend that a final PASS grade be achieved with a score of 100. In the absence of a large pilot study demonstrating standard normograms as is done for high-stakes testing, consensus of world renowned experts was obtained to delineate cut-off scores for the following four categories.

Category	Score
Novice	< 60
Advanced Beginner	60-79
Intermediate	80-99
Competent	100

Specific instructions marked by an asterisk (*) are provided for each of the tools.

Instructions: To administer the BSTAT, learners are asked to perform a complete diagnostic flexible bronchoscopy, while at all times stating what they are doing and where they are navigating in the airway. Thus, items 1, 2, 5, 6, and 7 are scored. They are then asked to go from the neutral position at the main carina to segments RB-4, 5, 6 and LB-8, 9, 10, and items 3 and 4 are scored. Items 8 and 9 are scored using the associated quiz images. Finally, item 10 is scored while the learner performs a BAL, brushing and mucosal biopsy. The BSTAT-TBLB/TBNA is also administered with a full diagnostic bronchoscopy, followed by a conventional TBNA and TBLB procedure (not necessarily all in the same patient, if assessment is being done in a patient). Items 5 and 10 are quiz-based images.

Bronchoscopy Skills and Tasks Assessment Tool (BSTAT)

- Items 1-10 may be scored separately.
- A passing score of 100 is expected to reflect competency.
- Scores <100 should initiate instructor-learner feedback
- Assessments may be performed in models or in patients.
- Knowledge of nomenclature (common language) for bronchoscopic findings can be assessed using the quiz. Recognition of findings can also be assessed during a bronchoscopic inspection, in which case instructors may prefer to use each quiz as a learning guide.
- The combined use of the 10 items pertains to technical skills needed to climb the learning curve from novice to competent bronchoscopist able to independently perform flexible bronchoscopy with lavage, brushing and endobronchial biopsy.
- This assessment tool is complementary to other methods of assessment such as practical approach exercises, checklists, logbooks of numbers of procedures performed, and outcomes.

§

Bronchoscopy Skills and Tasks Assessment Tool (BSTAT)

Learner: ______________________________ Training Year ____________

Faculty ______________________________ Date ____________

Educational Item* Items 1-10 each scored separately	**Satisfactory Yes/No**
1. Identification of Right sided anatomy (2 points each, target 20 points) ☐ RB1 apical ☐ RB2 posterior ☐ RB3 anterior ☐ RB4 lateral ☐ RB5 medial ☐ RB6 superior ☐ RB7 mediobasal ☐ RB8 anterobasal ☐ RB9 laterobasal ☐ RB10 posterobasal	Yes / No Score ____/20
2. Identification of Left sided anatomy (2 points each, target 16 points) ☐ LB1+2 apical/posterior ☐ LB3 anterior ☐ LB4 superior ☐ LB5 inferior ☐ LB6 superior ☐ LB8 anterobasal ☐ LB9 laterobasal ☐ LB10 posterobasal	Yes / No Score ____/16
3. Identify and enter RB 4+5+6 on demand (All three segments must be entered to earn 5 points, no partial points given, target 5 points) ☐ RB 4+5+6	Yes / No Score ____/5
4. Identify and enter LB 8+9+10 on demand (All three segments must be entered to earn 5 points, no partial points given, target 5 points) ☐ LB 8+9+10	Yes / No Score ____/5
5. Posture/Hand positions/Equipment safety (3 points each, target 9 points) ☐ Body posture ☐ Hand positions ☐ Equipment handling	Yes / No Score ____/9
6. Scope centered and kept in midline (5 points, no partial points given) ☐ Scope centered in airway lumen	Yes / No Score ____/5
7. Airway wall trauma avoided (5 points, no partial points given) ☐ Airway wall trauma avoided	Yes / No Score ____/5
8. Nomenclature: secretions descriptions (1 point each, target 10 points) ☐ Image 1 ☐ Image 2 ☐ Image 3 ☐ Image 4 ☐ Image 5 ☐ Image 6 ☐ Image 7 ☐ Image 8 ☐ Image 9 ☐ Image 10	Yes / No Score ____/10
9. Nomenclature: Mucosal descriptions (1 point each, target 10 points) ☐ Image 1 ☐ Image 2 ☐ Image 3 ☐ Image 4 ☐ Image 5 ☐ Image 6 ☐ Image 7 ☐ Image 8 ☐ Image 9 ☐ Image 10	Yes / No Score ____/10
10. Tasks: (5 points each, target 15 points) ☐ BAL ☐ Mucosal biopsy ☐ Brush	Yes / No Score ____/15

* The combined use of the 10 items pertains to technical skills needed to climb learning curve from novice to advanced beginner to intermediate to competent bronchoscopist able to perform flexible bronchoscopy with lavage, brushing and endobronchial biopsy independently.

FINAL GRADE PASS FAIL **SCORE** __________/100

Bstat Quiz Questions

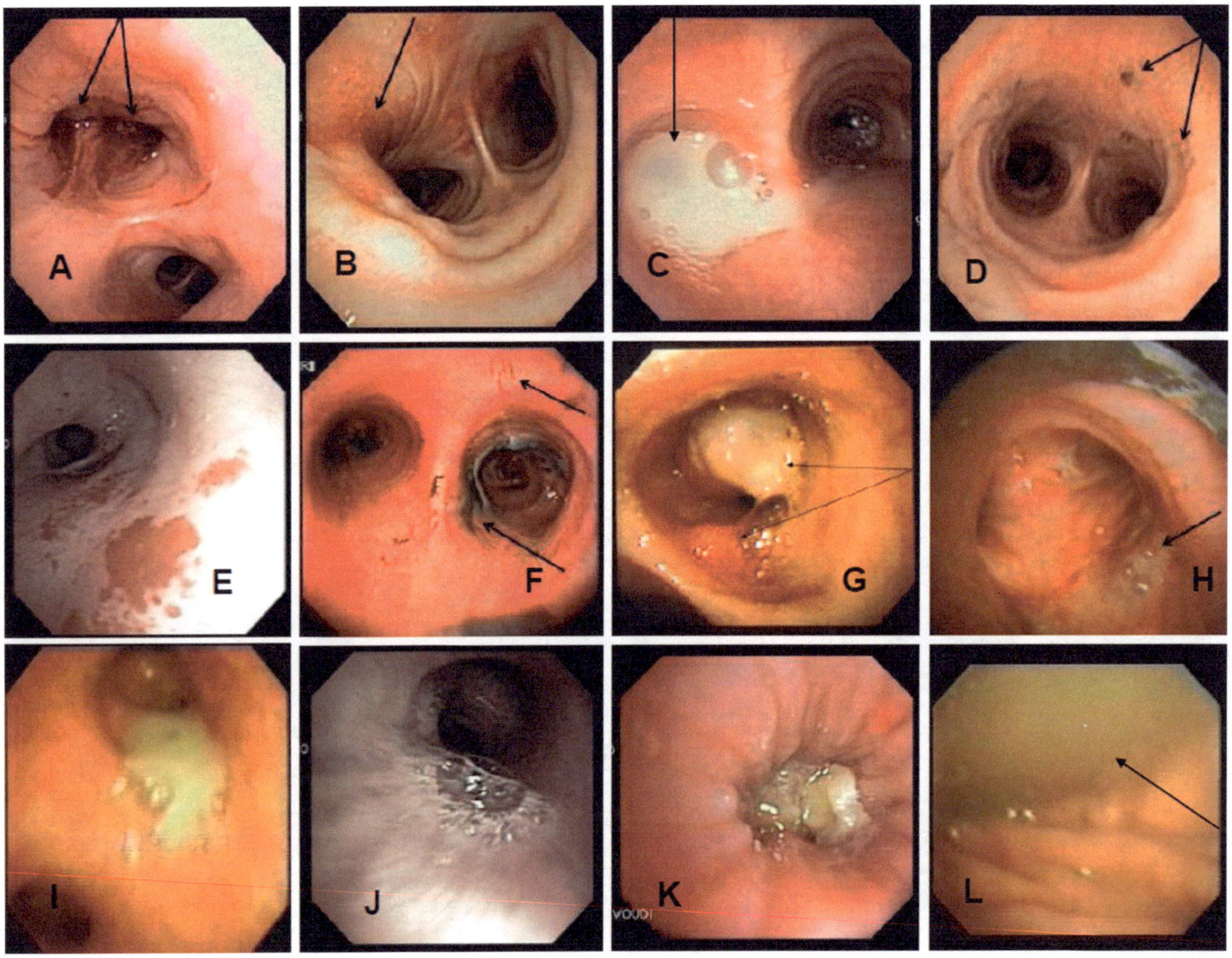

Item 8: Match the photo (A-L) to the corresponding 10 secretion descriptions (Only one response per description)

______ Sooty-burns	______ Bloody	______ Necrotic debris	______ Yellow purulent
______ White creamy	______ Normal clear	______ Tar-stained smoker's phlegm	______ Frothy covering TE fistula
______ Pink frothy edema	______ Scope trauma	NO RESPONSE	

BSTAT Quiz Questions

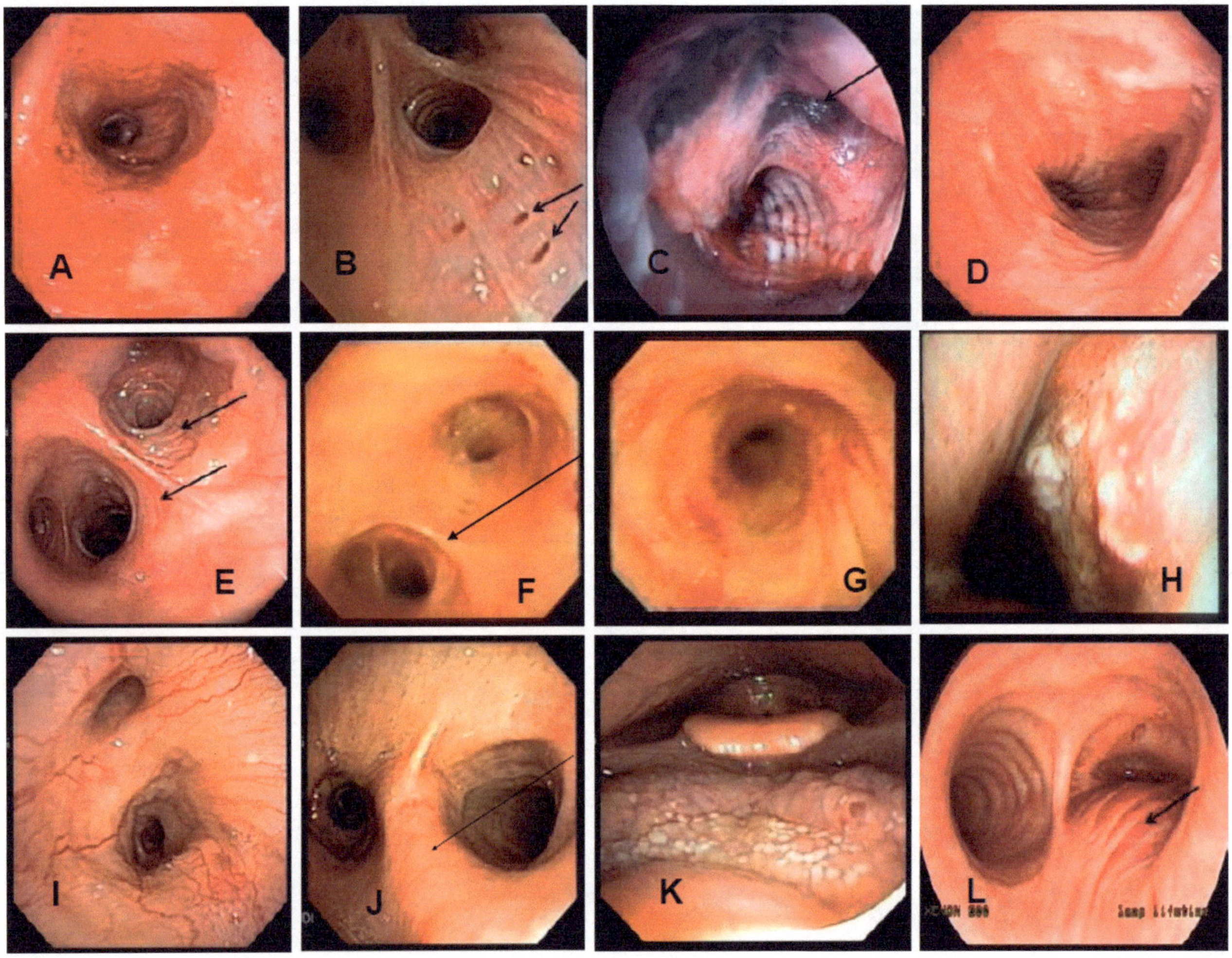

Item 9: Match the photo (A-L) to the corresponding 10 mucosal descriptions
(Only one response per description)

____________ Exophytic cancer	____________ Necrotic tracheitis	____________ Bronchial pits	____________ Chronic bronchitis
____________ Hypervascularity	____________ Tumor infiltrated carina	____________ Extrinsic compression	____________ Anthracosis
____________ Oral candidiasis	____________ Acute bronchitis	NO RESPONSE	

USER INSTRUCTIONS

Bronchoscopy Skills and Tasks Assessment Tool (BSTAT)

Educational Item* Items 1-10 each scored separately	**Satisfactory Yes/No**
1. Identification of Right sided anatomy (2 points each, target 20 points) ☐ RB1 apical ☐ RB2 posterior ☐ RB3 anterior ☐ RB4 lateral ☐ RB5medial ☐ RB6 superior ☐ RB7 mediobasal ☐ RB8 anterobasal ☐ RB9 laterobasal ☐ RB10 posterobasal *Each segment correctly identified AND entered scores TWO points.	Yes / No Score ____/20
2. Identification of Left sided anatomy (2 points each, target 16 points) ☐ LB1+2 apical/posterior ☐ LB3 anterior ☐ LB4 superior ☐ LB5 inferior ☐ LB6 superior ☐ LB8 anterobasal ☐ LB9 laterobasal ☐ LB10 posterobasal *Each segment correctly identified AND entered scores TWO points	Yes / No Score ____/16
3. Identify and enter RB 4+5+6 on demand (All three segments must be entered to earn 5 points, no partial points given, target 5 points) ☐ RB 4+5+6 * All THREE of these segments must be identified and entered correctly using appropriate flexion/extension of the bronchoscope in order to obtain FIVE points. No partial points are given. This is an "All or None" exercise.	Yes / No Score ____/5
4. Identify and enter LB 8+9+10 on demand (All three segments must be entered to earn 5 points, no partial points given, target 5 points) ☐ LB 8+9+10 All THREE of these segments must be identified and entered correctly using appropriate manipulation of the bronchoscope in order to obtain FIVE points. No partial points are given. This is an "All or None" exercise.	Yes / No Score ____/5
5. Posture/Hand positions/Equipment safety (3 points each, target 9 points) ☐ Body posture ☐ Hand positions ☐ Equipment handling *Procedures are taught different ways. In general however, students should be able to refrain from moving around the patient, they should avoid placing their hands into a patients eyes or exerting too much pressure onto a patient's head. The scope should be kept relatively straight, and should not be twisted at the insertion site. The hand holding the scope should be relaxed, and assistant should be able to easily access the hand being used to hold and manipulate accessory instruments. The bronchoscopist should be able to protect the scope from trauma (biting, slamming against a cart, dropping onto the floor). For each of the items, THREE points (or none) are given.	Yes / No Score ____/9

6. Scope centered and kept in midline (5 points, no partial points given) ☐ Scope centered in airway lumen In general, the scope should be kept centered so that it does not rub up against the airway wall. This is especially important when inserting the scope to the larynx, passing the vocal cords, and examining segmental bronchi. A scope that is not well-centered decreases overall visualization and may cause airway wall trauma or cough. If the scope is centered in the airway throughout most of the procedure, a score of FIVE points is achieved. No partial points are given. This is an "All or None" exercise.	Yes / No Score ____/5
7. Airway wall trauma avoided (5 points, no partial points given) ☐ Airway wall trauma avoided * In general, airway wall trauma causes erythema, swelling or cough. During the procedure, the scope should be kept "off the wall" using careful manipulation of the lateral as well as flexion/ extension function of the scope and appropriate identification and entry into segmental bronchi. If airway wall trauma is avoided during most of the procedure, a score of FIVE points is achieved. No partial points are given. This is an "All or None" exercise.	Yes / No Score ____/5
8. Nomenclature: secretions descriptions (1 point each, target 10 points) ☐ Sooty-burn ☐ Bloody ☐ Necrotic debris ☐ Yellow purulent ☐ White creamy ☐ Normal clear ☐ Tar-stained smokers phlegm ☐ Frothy covering TE fistula ☐ Pink frothy edema ☐ Scope trauma * This is a written test for which 1 point is given for each correct answer; to be used with associated slide-show.	Yes / No Score ____/10
9. Nomenclature: Mucosal descriptions (1 point each, target 10 points) ☐ Exophytic cancer ☐ Necrotic tracheitis ☐ Bronchial pits ☐ Chronic bronchitis ☐ Hypervascularity ☐ Tumor infiltrated carina ☐ Extrinsic compression ☐ Anthracosis ☐ Oral candidiasis ☐ Acute bronchitis *This is a written test for which 1 point is given for each correct answer; to be used with associated slide-show.	Yes / No Score ____/10
10. Tasks: (5 points each, target 15 points) ☐ BAL ☐ Mucosal biopsy ☐ Brush * This is an "All or None" exercise for which FIVE points are given to each of the 3 items if performed correctly. No partial points are given within each item.	Yes / No Score ____/15

* The combined use of these 10 items pertains to technical skills needed to climb learning curve from novice to advanced beginner to intermediate to competent bronchoscopist able to perform flexible bronchoscopy with BAL, brushing and mucosal biopsy.

FINAL GRADE PASS FAIL **SCORE** __________/100

BSTAT Quiz Answers

Bronchoscopy Skills and Tasks Answers...

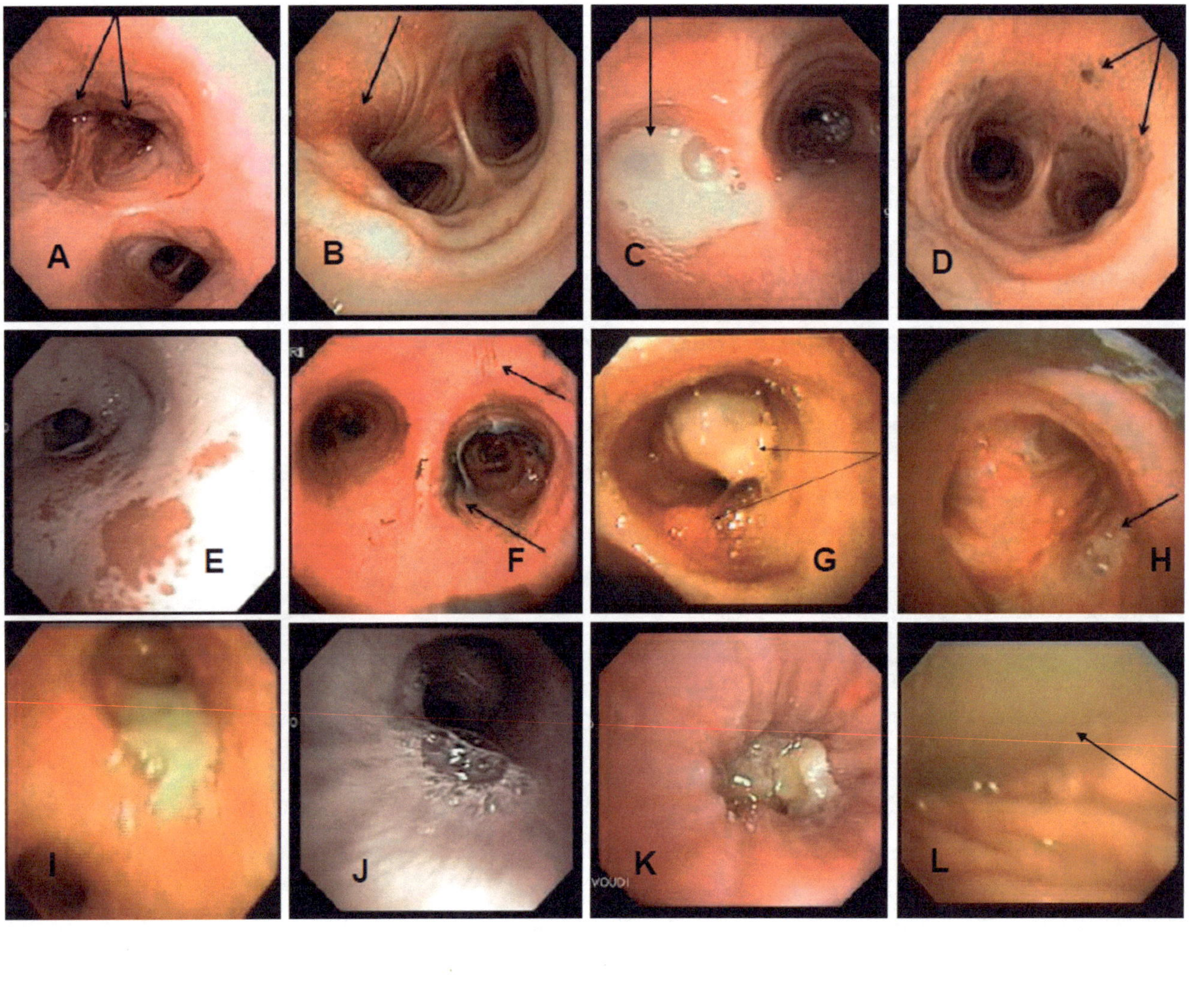

Item 8: Match the photo (A-L) to the corresponding 10 secretion descriptions (Only one response per description)

____F____ Sooty-burns	____A____ Bloody	____K____ Necrotic debris	____I____ Yellow purulent
____C____ White creamy	____J____ Normal clear	____D____ Tar-stained smoker's phlegm	____H____ Frothy covering TE fistula
____B____ Pink frothy edema	____E____ Scope trauma	NO RESPONSE	

Bronchoscopy Skills and Tasks Answers

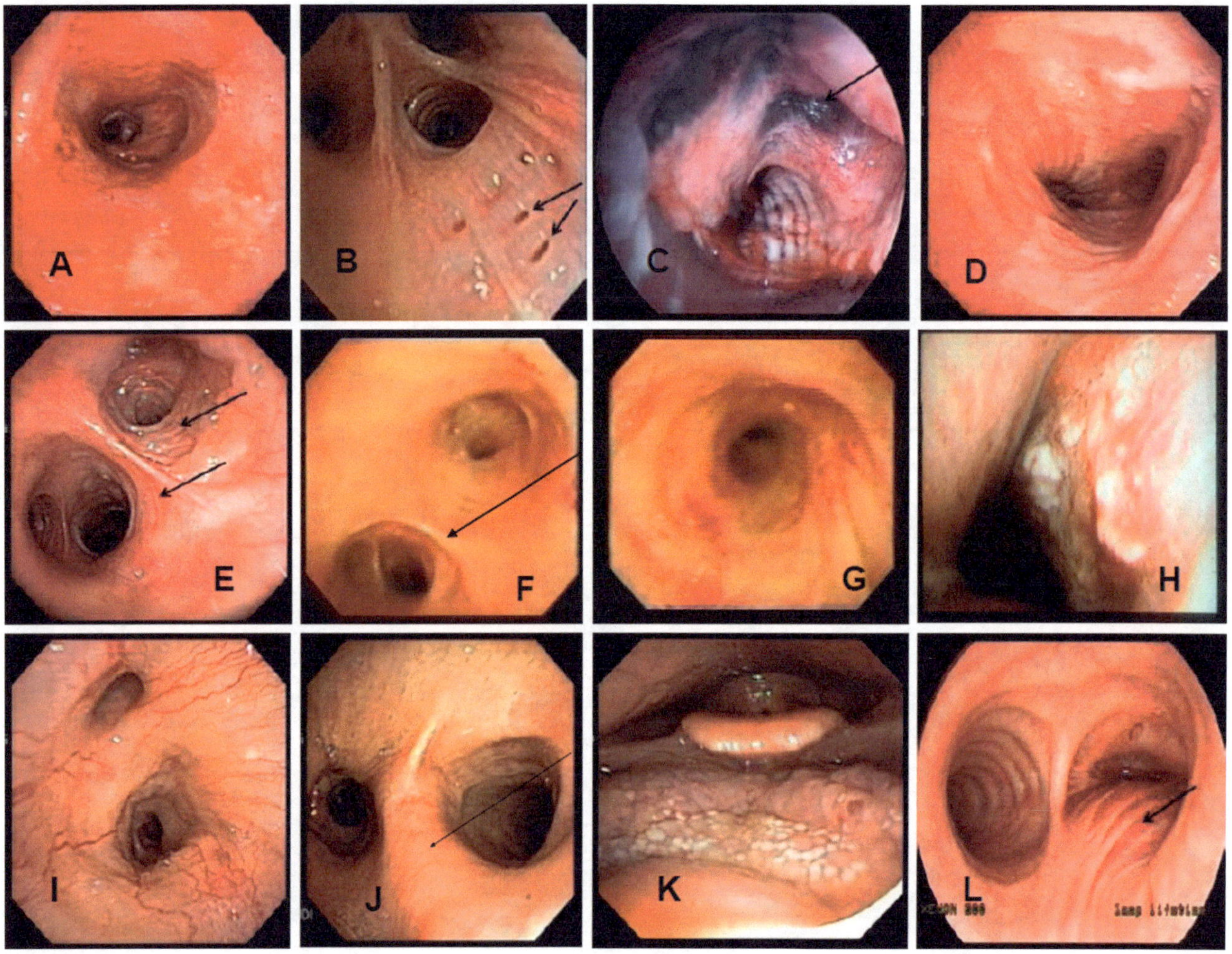

Item 9: Match the photo (A-L) to the corresponding 10 mucosal descriptions (Only one response per description)

____H____ Exophytic cancer	____D____ Necrotic tracheitis	____B____ Bronchial pits	____E____ Chronic bronchitis
____I____ Hypervascularity	____J____ Tumor infiltrated carina	____L____ Extrinsic compression	____C____ Anthracosis
____K____ Oral candidiasis	____A____ Acute bronchitis	NO RESPONSE	

Bronchoscopy Skills and Tasks TBLB/TBNA Assessment Tool (BSTAT-TBLB/TBNA)*

- Items 1-10 may be scored separately.
- A passing score of 100 is expected to reflect competency.
- Scores <100 should initiate instructor-learner feedback
- Assessments may be performed in models or in patients.
- Knowledge of nomenclature (common language) for bronchoscopic findings can be assessed using the quiz. Recognition of findings can also be assessed during a bronchoscopic inspection, in which case instructors may prefer to use each quiz as a learning guide.
- The combined use of the 10 items pertains to technical skills needed to climb the learning curve from novice to competent bronchoscopist able to independently perform flexible bronchoscopy with lavage, brushing and endobronchial biopsy.
- This assessment tool is complementary to other methods of assessment such as practical approach exercises, checklists, logbooks of numbers of procedures performed, and outcomes.

* While it is understood that some institutions may not perform conventional TBNA, we believe this skill should still be learned in case EBUS is unavailable. Institutions wishing to exclude training in conventional TBNA may choose to use only the TBLB portion of this assessment tool, using a passing score of 50 as a reflection of competency

§

Bronchoscopy Skills and Tasks Assessment Tool for Transbronchial Lung Biopsy and Transbronchial Needle Aspiration (BSTAT-TBLB/TBNA)

Learner: ______________________________ Training Year ______________

Faculty ______________________________ Date ______________

Educational Item* Items 1-10 each scored separately	**Satisfactory Yes/No**
1. TBLB: Airway inspection without trauma (no partial points) ☐ Complete inspection done properly	Yes / No Score ____/5
2. TBLB technique (no partial points) ☐ Wedge scope into target segment ☐ Visualize target with fluoroscopy ☐ Advance forceps under fluoroscopy guidance to target ☐ Open forceps at target ☐ Advance and close forceps at target ☐ Remove forceps from scope	Yes / No Score ____/10
3. TBLB Complications: Pneumothorax (no partial points) ☐ Perform panoramic view of hemithorax using fluoroscopy ☐ Recognize signs and symptoms ☐ Demonstrate easy access to small or large bore chest tube	Yes / No Score ____/10
4. TBLB: Complications: Bleeding (no partial points) ☐ Scope wedged into target segment ☐ Move patient into lateral decubitus safety position ☐ Access upper airway with oral suction ☐ Demonstrate access and use of bite block and endotracheal tube	Yes / No Score ____/10
5. TBLB: Decision making (5 points each, target score 15 points) ☐ Image 1 ☐ Image 2 ☐ Image 3	Yes / No Score ____/15
6. TBNA: Airway inspection and imaging interpretation (5 points each) ☐ Complete inspection done properly ☐ Imaging studies correctly interpreted	Yes / No Score ____/10
7. TBNA Technique - Jab (no partial points) ☐ Advance catheter towards target area ☐ Advance needle to target area without airway trauma ☐ Jab needle through airway wall at target region while scope is fixed at nose or mouth ☐ Move needle back and forth inside node while suctioning ☐ Release suction prior to needle withdrawal from target region ☐ Retract needle into the catheter ☐ Observe that needle is completely retracted inside catheter ☐ Withdraw catheter from scope	Yes / No Score ____/10
8. TBNA Technique-Hub against wall (no partial points) ☐ Advance catheter towards target area ☐ Touch catheter to target area without airway trauma ☐ Penetrate airway wall with needle while holding scope firmly ☐ Move needle back and forth inside node while suctioning ☐ Release suction prior to needle withdrawal from target region ☐ Retract needle into the catheter ☐ Observe that needle is completely retracted inside catheter ☐ Withdraw catheter from scope	Yes / No Score ____/10

9. TBNA Technique -Piggyback: (no partial points) ☐ Secure catheter and scope simultaneously with one hand ☐ Advance scope and catheter as a single unit to target region ☐ Penetrate airway wall at target region ☐ Move needle back and forth inside node while suctioning ☐ Release suction prior to needle withdrawal from target region ☐ Retract needle into the catheter ☐ Observe that needle is completely retracted inside catheter ☐ Withdraw catheter from scope	Yes / No Score ____/10
10. TBNA: Decision making: (5 points each, target 10 points) ☐ Image 4 ☐ Image 5	Yes / No Score ____/10

* Combined use of 10 items pertains to technical skills needed to climb learning curve from novice to competent bronchoscopist able to perform flexible bronchoscopy with TBLB and TBNA independently.

FINAL GRADE PASS FAIL **SCORE** __________/100

TBLB Stat Quiz

BSTAT TBLB-TBNA Questions

NAME ______________________

ITEM 5: Choose **One** best answer for each question

1. The target region is most likely (A) RB1, (B) RB6, (C) RB9, (D) RB10,

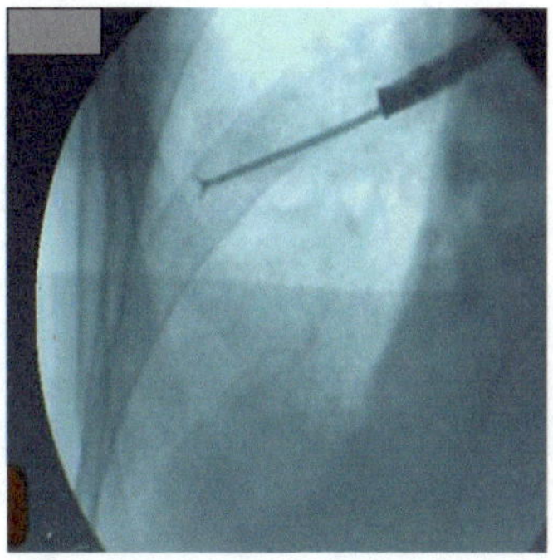

Answer ________

2. The target region is the (A) apical-posterior segment left upper lobe, (B) Lingula, (C) Right upper lobe

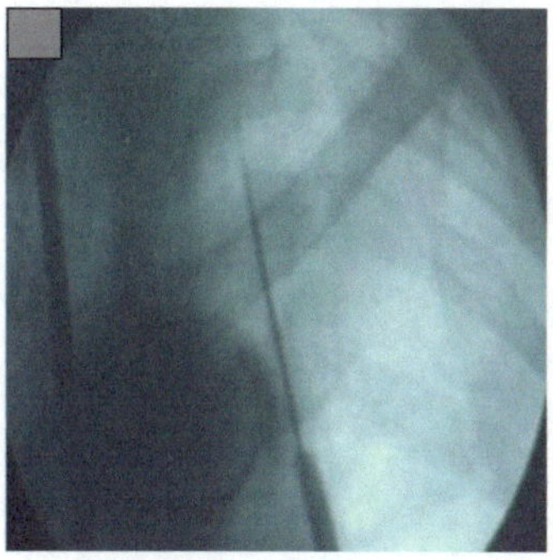

Answer ________

3. Which region should be biopsied in this immuno- suppressed patient with suspected fungal disease ?

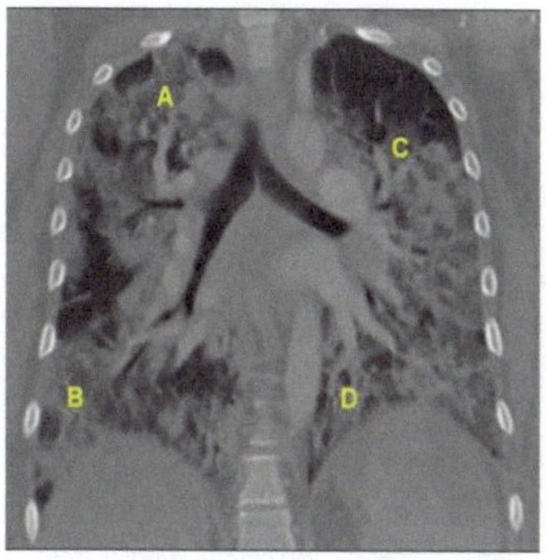

Answer ________

ITEM 10: Choose **One** best answer for each question

4. During conventional TBNA, which of the following lymph nodes will likely offer the highest diagnostic yield for nonsmall cell lung cancer ?

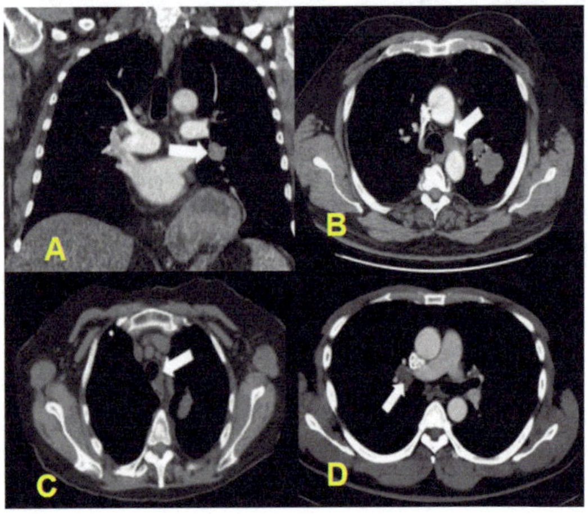

Answer ________

5. Where is the node located (needle insertion site E, F,G, or H)?

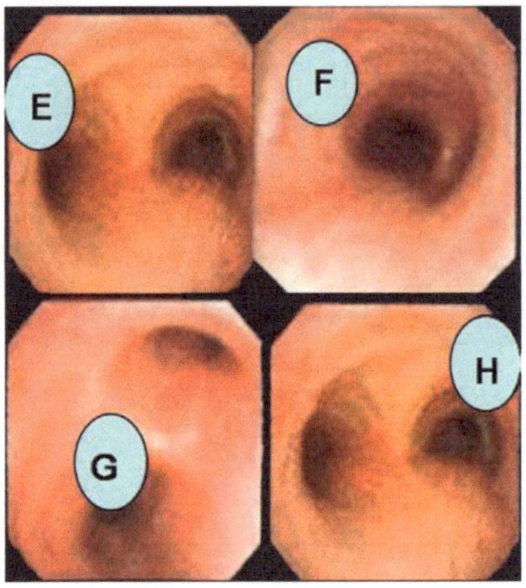

Answer ________

USER INSTRUCTIONS

Bronchoscopy Skills and Tasks Assessment Tool, for Transbronchial Lung Biopsy and Transbronchial Needle Aspiration (BSTAT-TBLB/TBNA)

Educational Item* Items 1-10 each scored separately	**Satisfactory Yes/No**
1. TBLB: Airway inspection without trauma (no partial points) ☐ Complete inspection done properly *It goes without saying that the student should be able to perform inspection bronchoscopy and be able to identify and enter all bronchial segments.	Yes / No Score ____/5
2. TBLB technique (no partial points) ☐ Wedge scope into target segment ☐ Visualize target with fluoroscopy ☐ Advance forceps under fluoroscopy guidance to target ☐ Open forceps at target ☐ Advance and close forceps at target ☐ Remove forceps from scope *Many techniques exist for TBLB, but the instructor should focus on certain universal principles. The student should be able to wedge and unwedge the scope, and go through the various motions for TBLB including use of expiration and inspiration. Proper use of fluoroscopy requires a passing grade on the fluoroscopy test. Communication is key with instructions such as open and close forceps. If all six steps are completed satisfactorily, the student receives 10 points.	Yes / No Score ____/10
3. TBLB Complications: Pneumothorax (no partial points) ☐ Perform panoramic view of hemithorax using fluoroscopy ☐ Recognize signs and symptoms ☐ Demonstrate easy access to small or large bore chest tube *The student should be able to demonstrate the ability to respond quickly to this adverse event. Team communication is key, and the instructor should ascertain that the student is able to give appropriate instructions to nursing staff.	Yes / No Score ____/10
4. TBLB: Complications: Bleeding (no partial points) ☐ Scope wedged into target segment ☐ Move patient into lateral decubitus safety position ☐ Access upper airway with oral suction ☐ Demonstrate access and use of bite block and endotracheal tube *The student should be able to demonstrate the ability to respond quickly to this adverse event. Team communication is key, and the instructor should ascertain that the student is able to give appropriate instructions to nursing staff.	Yes / No Score ____/10
5. TBLB: Decision making (5 points each , target score 15 points) ☐ Image 1 ☐ Image 2 ☐ Image 3 *The written test also serves as the answer sheet; to be used with associated slide-show. Tests should be collected. Students can be given their scores, but should not be provided with the correct answers so that they can take the test at a later date	Yes / No Score ____/15

6. TBNA: Airway inspection and imaging interpretation (5 points each) ☐ Complete inspection done properly ☐ Imaging studies correctly interpreted Imaging studies should be reviewed prior to bronchoscopy. Instructor should be certain that the student can justify the procedure and has formulated a plan.	Yes / No Score ____/10
7. TBNA Technique - Jab (no partial points) ☐ Advance catheter towards target area ☐ Advance needle to target area without airway trauma ☐ Jab needle through airway wall at target region while scope is fixed at nose or mouth ☐ Move needle back and forth inside node while suctioning ☐ Release suction prior to needle withdrawal from target region ☐ Retract needle into the catheter ☐ Observe that needle is completely retracted inside catheter ☐ Withdraw catheter from scope *While there are many ways to perform TBNA these universal principles and instructions are well described by experts. The student should understand these principles and be able to perform each of the three techniques because each one may be necessary in a different setting. The student should be using appropriate safety measures in regards to needle in, needle out instructions, handling the needle catheter, and while withdrawing the catheter from the scope. No partial points are given for any of the techniques.	Yes / No Score ____/10
8. TBNA Technique-Hub against wall (no partial points) ☐ Advance catheter towards target area ☐ Touch catheter to target area without airway trauma ☐ Penetrate airway wall with needle while holding scope firmly ☐ Move needle back and forth inside node while suctioning ☐ Release suction prior to needle withdrawal from target region ☐ Retract needle into the catheter ☐ Observe that needle is completely retracted inside catheter ☐ Withdraw catheter from scope	Yes / No Score ____/10
9. TBNA Technique -Piggyback: (no partial points) ☐ Secure catheter and scope simultaneously with one hand ☐ Advance scope and catheter as a single unit to target region ☐ Penetrate airway wall at target region ☐ Move needle back and forth inside node while suctioning ☐ Release suction prior to needle withdrawal from target region ☐ Retract needle into the catheter ☐ Observe that needle is completely retracted inside catheter ☐ Withdraw catheter from scope	Yes / No Score ____/10
10. TBNA: Decision making: (5 points each, target 10 points) ☐ Image 4 ☐ Image 5 *The written test serves as the answer sheet; to be used with associated slide-show. Tests should be collected. Learners are given their scores, but should not be provided with the correct answers so that they can take the test at a later date	Yes / No Score ____/10

* The combined use of these 10 items pertains to technical skills needed to climb learning curve from novice to advanced beginner to intermediate to competent bronchoscopist able to perform flexible bronchoscopy with transbronchial lung biopsy and transbronchial needle aspiration independently.

FINAL GRADE PASS FAIL **SCORE** __________/100

TBLB Stat Answer

BSTAT TBLB-TBNA Answers

ITEM 5: Choose **One** best answer for each question

1. The target region is most likely (A) RB1, (B) RB6, (C) RB9, (D) RB10,

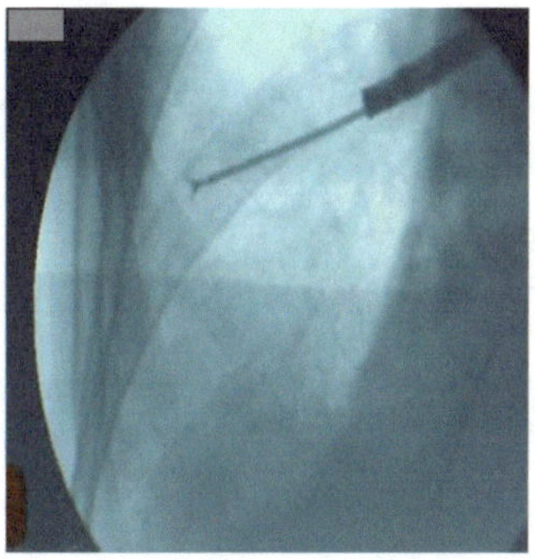

Answer ____C____

2. The target region is the (A) apical-posterior segment left upper lobe, (B) Lingula, (C) Right upper lobe

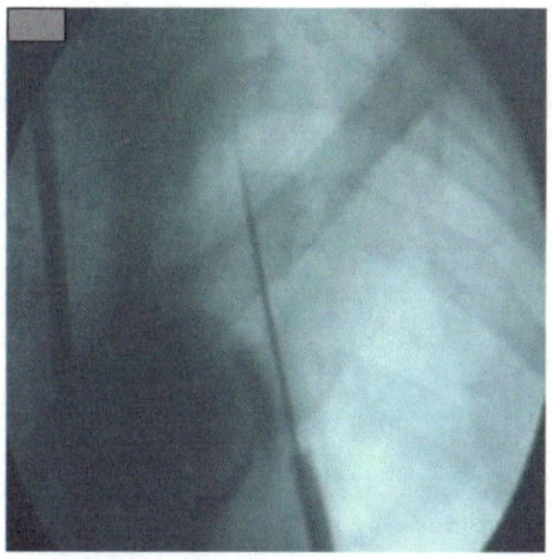

Answer ____A____

3. Which region should be biopsied in this immuno- suppressed patient with suspected fungal disease ?

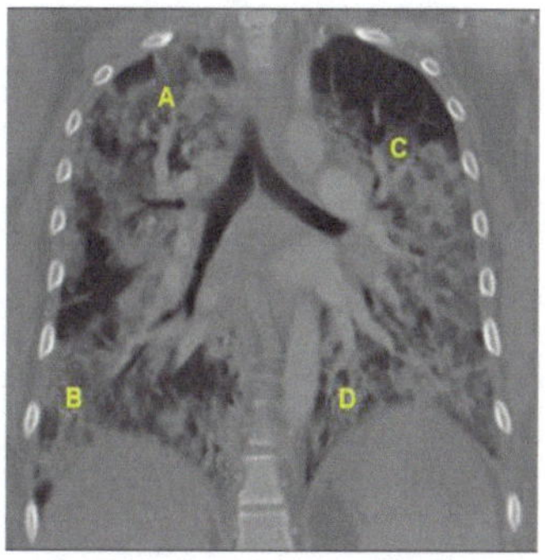

Answer ____B____

ITEM 10: Choose **One** best answer for each question

4. During conventional TBNA, which of the following lymph nodes will likely offer the highest diagnostic yield for nonsmall cell lung cancer ?

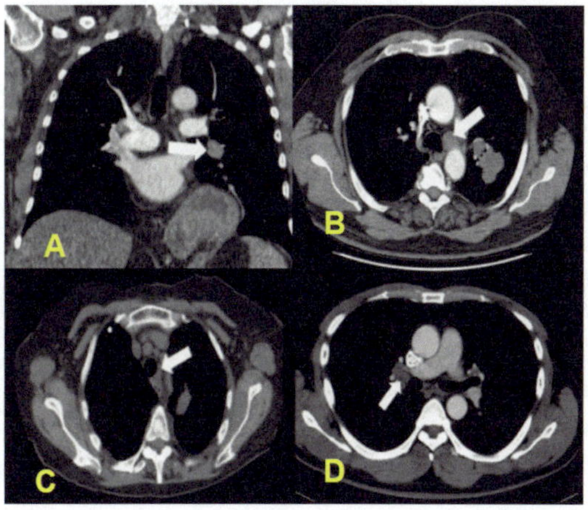

Answer ____B____

5. Where is the node located (needle insertion site E, F,G, or H)?

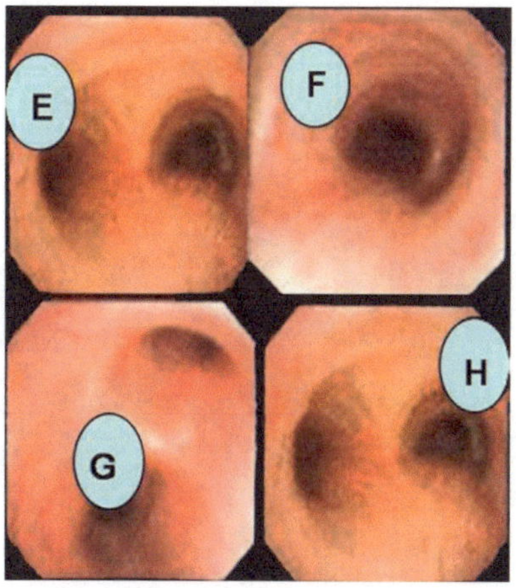

Answer ____E____

Bronchoscopy Self Assessment Tool (BSAT)

- Items 1-10 may be assessed separately.
- There is no "passing score" for this assessment tool.
- The purpose of this assessment tool is to initiate instructor-learner feedback and to identify areas that warrant further reinforcement.
- Assessments may be performed in models or in patients.
- Assessments may be performed before and after a series of training sessions or clinical procedures.
- This assessment tool is complementary to other methods of assessment such as BSTAT and BSTAT-TBLB/TBNA, EBUS-STAT, practical approach exercises, checklists, logbooks of numbers of procedures performed, and outcomes.

§

USER INSTRUCTIONS

Bronchoscopy Self Assessment Tool (BSAT)

The purpose of this assessment tool is to provide bidirectional feedback between learner and instructor. There are no wrong answers. Well performed, this interaction will allow opportunities to ascertain strengths and weaknesses of a training program and educational methodologies. In addition, an open discussion will allow both learner and instructor to identify the learner's zones of proximal development and reflective capacity[1]. Educators may wish to ask learners to complete the BSAT prior to the encounter, and to then review each element of the questionnaire with the learner in order to identify which areas might warrant additional concentration.

1	2	3	4	5
Not comfortable		Comfortable		Very comfortable

1. I am able to identify airway anatomy ___
2. I am able to identify airway mucosal abnormalities ___
3. I am able to describe secretions and other airway abnormalities ___
4. I am able to maneuver the flexible bronchoscope ___
5. I am able to do a BAL through the flexible scope ___
6. I am able to use a brush through the flexible bronchoscope ___
7. I am able to use biopsy forceps through the scope ___
8. I am able to perform transbronchial lung biopsy ___
9. I am able to perform conventional transbronchial needle aspiration ___
10. I now feel comfortable performing this case in a patient ___

Anatomy Abnormalities Technique Equipment Interpretation of findings

I would like to learn more about (circle all that apply above)

1	2	3	4	5
Poor	Below average	Average	Good	Excellent

Using the above scale please rate your training as (please circle one of the above)

I have the following comments

[1] The constructivist psychologist Lev Vygotsky (1896-1934) believed that learning and development depend on social interaction. Focusing primarily on how children learn, he described a zone of proximal development (ZPD) as "the distance between the actual development level as determined by independent problem solving and the level of potential development as determined through problem solving under adult guidance or in collaboration with more capable peers" (L.S. Vygotsky: *Mind in Society: Development of Higher Psychological Processes*, p. 86, John-Steiner, Cole, Scribner, and Souberman Editors, Harvard University Press ,1980). Tinsley and Lebak expanded on this theory, describing a zone of reflective capacity in which adults increased their ability for critical reflection through feedback, analyses, and evaluation of one another's work in a collaborative working environment (Lebak, K. & Tinsley, R. Can inquiry and reflection be contagious? Science teachers, students, and action research. Journal of Science Teacher Education;2010:21;953-970).

Essential Flexible Bronchoscopist©
Post-tests

Post-tests are multiple choice, single BEST answer.

While many programs consider 70% correct responses a passing grade, the learner's "target" score should be 100%.

Passing grades on each of the post-tests are desirable and should be noted on the BEP Program completion checklist.

The Essential Flexible Bronchoscopist© is comprised of six modules, each with a module-specific competency-oriented list of learning objectives. There are a total of 186 multiple choice question sets. These are also viewable on line in fourteen languages at the Bronchoscopy International website (see, www.Bronchoscopy.org) and downloadable from https://bronchoscopy.org/essential-bronchoscopist/. Books are available for purchase in paperback and Kindle versions on Amazon.

Information pertains to major topics represented in traditional textbooks of bronchoscopy, including anatomy and airway abnormalities, patient preparation, indications, contraindications, complications, techniques and solutions to technical difficulties, primary and metastatic lung cancer, infections, tracheal stenosis and other airway disorders of benign etiology, anesthesia and moderate sedation, medications, informed consent, patient safety issues, equipment maintenance, history of bronchoscopy, bronchioloalveolar lavage, endobronchial biopsy, washings, brushings, conventional transbronchial needle aspiration, bronchoscopic lung biopsy, and basics of interventional bronchoscopy.

The aim of **The Essential Flexible Bronchoscopist©** is to enhance the learner's progress along the learning curve from novice to competent practitioner. To encourage interactive learning and communication among peers, many question/answer sets are intentionally written so that a correct response is not readily apparent.

At the end of each module is a set of ten post-test questions. These are best answered before moving to the next module. None are meant to serve as high stakes tests, but rather as low-stakes continuing self-learning assessments that help document the progressive acquisition of knowledge needed for the safe and competent practice of bronchoscopy. Question/answer sets of **The Essential Flexible Bronchoscopist©** can be used during didactic lectures or during pretest-posttest sessions at regional meetings. The reader is encouraged to answer these questions AFTER reading the corresponding module. An honor system is assumed in regards to viewing provided answers to these post-tests on the following pages.

The Essential Flexible Bronchoscopist©
Module I Post-test Questions

Q1: In addition to Shigeto Ikeda and Gustav Killian, a critical figure in the history of bronchoscopy education and practice is:

A. Sir William Osler
B. *Chevalier* Jackson
C. Laennec
D. William Harvey

Q2: Which of the following should be required of every patient undergoing flexible bronchoscopy?

A. Coagulation profile
B. Serum chemistries, especially blood urea nitrogen and creatinine
C. Electrocardiogram
D. Review of known or suspected allergies to medications

Q3: Among which of the following settings has flexible bronchoscopy been shown to be of greatest value ?

A. Patient with hemoptysis and a nonlocalizing chest radiograph
B. Patient with smoking history, cough, weight loss, and lung mass on chest radiograph
C. Patient with a peripheral lung nodule less than 1 cm in diameter
D. Prior to thoracentesis in a patient with suspected malignant pleural effusion

Q4: Scenarios where airway management might be difficult and could therefore warrant bronchoscopic assistance include each of the following except ?

A. An 18-year-old male with status asthmaticus and altered mental status who just vomited his dinner.
B. Pregnant 30-year-old obese woman with third degree facial burns.
C. Edentulous male undergoing cardiopulmonary resuscitation
D. Elderly trauma victim wearing neck brace

Q5: In regards to handling the flexible bronchoscope, which of the below is considered correct technique?

A. Moving the scope between the left hand and the right hand during the procedure.
B. Keeping the scope in the middle of the airway lumen as much as possible during the procedure.
C. Twisting the scope at its insertion point at the mouth or the nares in order to direct it into an upper lobe bronchus.
D. Moving the thumb downwards to flex the distal aspect of the insertion tube.

Q6: Which of the following statements pertaining to local anesthetics is false ?

A. Lidocaine and Bupivicaine are both esters
B. Amides, as Mepivicaine, as well as esters, such as Tetracaine can cause laryngeal edema.
C. Bilateral nasal administration of anesthetic causes partial posterior pharyngeal anesthesia by affecting the Sphenopalatine nerve fibers.
D. Administration of lidocaine with epinephrine can decrease swelling of the nasal mucosal membranes.
E. Many side effects of topical anesthetics are dose related, but anaphylaxis is not.

Q7: Which of the following statements about upper airway anatomy is incorrect?

A. In adults, the glottic opening (also called the rima glottides) is more narrow than the cricoid.
B. An omega epiglottis is elongated, curved and is seen in adults but also in many infants.
C. The arytenoid cartilages lie superior to the corniculate cartilages at the posterior commissure of the larynx.
D. The adult trachea cross-sectional area, usually about 2.8 cm^2, increases with age
E. The recurrent laryngeal nerve supplies motor and sensory innervation of the intrinsic muscles of the larynx.

Q8: Which of the following adverse effects of bronchoscopy is probably most frequent ?

A. Biopsy-induced pneumothorax
B. Bronchoalveolar lavage induced hypoxemia
C. Pain, discomfort or anxiety during insertion of the bronchoscope and passage into the lower airways
D. Cardiac arrhythmias

Q9: Which of the following statements about the trachea is incorrect?

A. The cervical segment (extrathoracic) ends at the manubrium and encompasses about the first six tracheal rings.
B. The U-shaped trachea is probably the most frequent shape found.
C. A man's cross sectional tracheal area is usually about 40 percent larger than a woman's.
D. Saber sheath tracheas have a small transverse diameter, which means that the distance between the left and right lateral walls of the trachea is short.
E. In women, the lower limit of normal for transverse and sagittal diameters is about 10 mm.

Q10: Which of the following statements about radiation exposure during fluoroscopy is correct?

A. The patient's radiation exposure is increased as the anode tube is placed closer to the patient.
B. The bronchoscopist's radiation exposure makes wearing a protective lead garment unnecessary.
C. The patient's radiation exposure increase when the anode tube is further from the patient.
D. Radiation exposure is a measure of resolution, and can be adjusted by changing the size of the image on the fluoroscopy screen.

The Essential Flexible Bronchoscopist©
Module II Post-test Questions

Q1: Which of the following parts of a bronchoscope is most easily damaged?

A. The universal cord
B. The eyepiece or video control handle
C. The insertion tube
D. The control handle

Q2: Which of the following drugs can be safely used for effective topical anesthesia in a patient with an allergy to Lidocaine?

A. Atropine
B. Fentanyl
C. Tetracaine
D. Glycopyrolate

Q3: Dynamic bronchoscopy might be most helpful in patients with:

A. Suspected tuberculosis and upper lobe infiltrates
B. Suspected tracheobronchomalacia
C. A large obstructing endobronchial lesion noted on computed tomography scan
D. Ipsilateral lung mass and pleural effusion

Q4: Which of the following best helps prevent obstruction by dried secretions in patients with indwelling Montgomery T-tubes?

A. Placing the proximal part of the tube within 1 centimeter of the vocal cords
B. Keeping the external limb of the T-tube capped, except for suctioning.
C. Scheduling frequent and routine flexible bronchoscopy for suctioning
D. Keeping the external limb of the T-tube uncapped.

Q5: All of the following statements about flexible bronchoscopy in the intensive care unit setting are correct EXCEPT ?

A. Bronchoscopy can be helpful to remove secretions in mechanically ventilated patents.
B. Bronchoscopy can help resolve radiographic lobar atelectasis in mechanically ventilated patients.
C. Bronchoscopy should be routinely used instead of chest percussion and tracheal aspiration to remove secretions in intubated patients.
D. When scoping through the mouth, a bite block is essential to prevent scope damage, even in patients who are intubated orally.

Q6: Which of the following anatomic descriptions is correct?

A. The trachea extends from C6 to T5, in a downward and backward direction, and, near the tracheal bifurcation, deviates slightly to right.
B. The trachea extends from C6 to T5, in a downward and forward direction, and, near the tracheal bifurcation, deviates slightly to right
C. The trachea extends from C6 to T5, in a downward and backward direction, with the thyroid gland surrounding the anterolateral portion between the fourth and sixth cartilage rings.
D. The trachea extends from C6 to T5, in a downward and backward direction, with the thyroid gland surrounding the anterolateral portion between the first and third cartilage rings.

Q7: Viewing the vocal cords from below might be useful in all of the following cases EXCEPT?

A. To exclude a peristomal or subglottic source of bleeding in a patient with a tracheostomy.
B. To fully evaluate laryngeal function in a patient with a tracheostomy being decanulated.
C. To examine the subglottis and vocal cord function in a patient with suspected tracheal stenosis and a tracheostomy.
D. To remove subglottic granulation tissue using laser

Q8: Once in the airway, the flexible bronchoscope:

A. Occupies less than 5% of the normal airway diameter
B. Results in increased functional capacity, especially if there is also an endotracheal tube in place
C. Decreases airway resistance, especially if there is also an endotracheal tube in place
D. Occupies more than 20% of the normal airway diameter

Q9: High level disinfection does all of the following EXCEPT?

A. Inactivate all bacterial spores.
B. Inactivate all fungi
C. Destroy all viruses
D. Destroy all vegetative organisms.

Q10: Which of the following best describes a complex tracheal stricture?

A. Circumferential narrowing 3 cm below the vocal cords, extending along a distance of 2, without associated tracheomalacia.
B. Partially circumferential web-like stricture 3 cm below the vocal cords along the anterior wall of the trachea in a site of previous and well healed tracheostomy.
C. Bottleneck stricture 2 cm below the cords with asymmetric narrowing of the trachea and a second partial web at the distal margin of the bottleneck stenosis.
D. Circumferential narrowing of the trachea to 3 mm by fibrous tissue 2 cm below the vocal cords, extending along a distance of 0.5 cm.

The Essential Flexible Bronchoscopist©
Module III Post-test Questions

Q1: Which of the following best describes Midazolam?

A. Ten times more potent than diazepam
B. Sedation and anxiolysis usually occurs within 2 minutes of administration
C. Complete recovery of motor performance and consciousness often takes two hours
D. Risk for apnea is greatest when used alone compared to when used with other sedating agents.
E. Larger doses can cause seizures even in healthy patients

Q2: Repeated trauma to the larynx during attempts at bronchoscopically-assisted endotracheal intubation most likely to cause which of the following?

A. Laryngospasm, vomiting, and cardiac arrhythmias
B. Hoarseness, vocal cord paralysis, and arytenoid luxation
C. Laryngeal edema, aspiration, and fever
D. Pain, gagging, and diarrhea

Q3: When using Gluteraldehyde for high-level disinfection, a 10-minute immersion results in which of the following?

A. 50% eradication of mycobacteria
B. 85% eradication of mycobacteria
C. 99.8% eradication of mycobacteria
D. Complete eradication of mycobacteria

Q4: All of the following statements about scattered radiation are correct EXCEPT?

A. It is caused by increased voltage
B. It can be reduced by decreasing the anode tube milliamperage
C. It decreases the quality of the fluoroscopic image.
D. It is caused by increased tissue thickness

Q5: All of the following statements about topical Lidocaine are true EXCEPT?

A. The maximum dose recommended for flexible bronchoscopy is about 300 mg.
B. Systemic effects include restlessness, seizures, numbness, and hypotension.

C. It is less potent but longer acting than Tetracaine.
D. Peak concentration is usually reached within 30 minutes of airway application.

Q6: Which of the following statements best relates to patients with a saber-sheath trachea?

A. It may be found in up to 5 percent of elderly men.
B. The majority of patients with saber sheath trachea also have asthma
C. It is characterized by an increased transverse distance and decreased sagittal diameter of the trachea.
D. Differential diagnosis might include extrinsic compression, relapsing polychondritis, wegener's Granulomatosis, and Klebsiella Rhinoscleromata.

Q7: All of the following statements describing the "proper" way to dictate or write a bronchoscopy note are correct EXCEPT?

A. Consistently use the same concise and precise terminology.
B. Tell a story that everyone can read and understand the same way.
C. Consistently comment on airway patency, mucosal appearances, secretions, and location of specimens obtained.
D. Referring to the amount and effects of conscious sedation can usually be avoided.

Q8: The bronchus intermedius usually measures:

A. Less than 1.0 cm.
B. More than 2.5 cm.
C. Between 1.0 and 2.5 cm.
D. It is a misnomer because it immediately becomes the middle lobe and lower lobe bronchus.

Q9: All of the following statements about bronchoalveolar lavage are true EXCEPT?

A. Delayed onset fever, chills and myalgias are best treated with an antipyretic or other anti-inflammatory medication.
B. Radiographic infiltrates in the area of lavage are rarely visible after the procedure.
C. BAL may cause or increase hypoxemia
D. Careful technique is essential to obtain a true alveolar sample rather than a simple bronchial wash.

Q10: Which of the following statements about oral airways is MOST correct?

A. They help keep the scope in the midline, facilitating exposure of laryngeal structures.
B. They help maintain an open pharynx and larynx.
C. They prevent the patient from biting the bronchoscope.
D. They facilitate maneuverability of the scope and endotracheal intubation.

The Essential Flexible Bronchoscopist©
Module IV Post-test Questions

Q1: The average internal diameter of the left or right main bronchi, is about:

A. 5 -10 mm
B. 10-16 mm
C. 14-18 mm
D. 12-20 mm

Q2: Endobronchial metastases are unlikely in which of the following illness?

A. Colon cancer
B. Malignant melanoma
C. Gastric cancer
D. Breast cancer
E. Renal carcinoma

Q3: LC-1 corresponds to which of the following?

A. The minor carina between the lingula and the anterior segment of the upper division bronchus
B. The minor carina between the lingual and the apical segment of the upper division bronchus
C. The minor carina between the lingula and the lower lobe bronchus
D. The minor carina between the superior segment and the lower lobe bronchus

Q4: All of the following statements about bronchoalveolar lavage are true EXCEPT?

A. Cellular and noncellular components from the epithelial surfaces of the lower respiratory tract are recovered.
B. A 100 ml lavage samples approximately 10×10^6 alveoli
C. Fluid return is decreased in smokers and in the elderly
D. Procedures should be atraumatic, harmonious and result in no more than 10% bronchial squamous cells
E. It is appropriate to call BAL a "bronchioloalveolar lavage".

Q5: Generally accepted precautions for bronchoscopy in patients with thrombocytopenia include all of the following EXCEPT?

A. Administration of IVIG infusions for patients with Idiopathic Thrombocytopenic Purpura.
B. Platelet transfusions to increase platelet count so that it is at least greater than 20,000, and higher if biopsies are being performed.

C. Considering passage through the mouth (using a bite-block of course).
D. Bronchoscopy, even without biopsy, should be avoided, especially if patients have severe thrombocytopenia (counts below 20,000 platelets)

Q6: The nomenclature RC-2 corresponds to which of the following?

A. The minor carina between RB 2 and the Bronchus Intermedius.
B. The minor carina between RB 4, 5 and the lower lobe bronchus.
C. The minor carina between RB 6 and the bronchus intermedius.
D. The minor carina between RB 6 and the lower lobe bronchus.

Q7: Which of the following airway abnormalities is least likely to be due to chronic bronchitis?

A. Mucosal pitting.
B. Band formation and traction of longitudinal fibers.
C. Erythema and pallor.
D. Raised red areas of mucosal thickening and edema.

Q8: In a 62-year-old patient with cough, weight loss, pleural effusion, volume loss, and a suspected history of tuberculosis, bronchoscopy might be helpful for which of the following?

A. To discover possible bronchial strictures that might help explain the radiographic images.
B. To obtain specimens for diagnostic purposes.
C. To help exclude other potential diagnoses such as cancer.
D. All of the above.
E. None of the above. The patient should undergo thoracentesis or closed-needle pleural biopsy

Q9: Which of the following endobronchial findings best describes early superficial invasive cancer ?

A. Pale mucosa with lack of luster.
B. Red or granular lesions with increased friability.
C. Easy friability
D. Answers a and b
E. Answers a and c.

Q10: Which of the following anatomic structures lies directly adjacent to the anterior wall of the bronchus intermedius at the level of the take off of the right upper lobe bronchus?

A. The right pulmonary artery.
B. The right pulmonary vein.
C. The right pulmonary artery and pulmonary vein.
D. The esophagus
E. The thoracic duct.

The Essential Flexible Bronchoscopist©
Module V Post-test Questions

Q1: Which of the following nomenclatures pertain to the left lower lobe posterobasal segment, and the carina between the left upper lobe and left lower lobe bronchus?

A. LB 8 and LC-2
B. LB 10 and LC-2
C. LB 9 and LC-2
D. None of the above

Q2: A small malignant endobronchial abnormality is noted in the bronchus intermedius 0.5 cm beyond the right upper lobe bronchial orifice. Transcarinal needle aspirations are positive. CT scans reveal no other organ involvement. Which of the following best describes this patient's clinical TNM stage?

A. T3 N1 M0
B. T3 N2 M0
C. T2 N2 M0
D. T1 N2 M0
E. None of the above

Q3: Which of the following best describes the safety position during bronchoscopy?

A. Turning the patient unto the left position to facilitate suctioning.
B. Turning the patient onto the lateral decubitus position, bleeding side down in case of bronchoscopically-induced bleeding.
C. Turning the patient unto the lateral decubitus position, left side down, in case of vomiting during bronchoscopy.
D. Tilting the bed into the reverse Trendelenberg position in case of bronchoscopically-induced bleeding.

Q4: Which of the following best explains why airway lacerations and tracheoesophageal fistulas are easily missed during bronchoscopic examination?

A. Airway mucosa might swell and easily obliterate the lesion.
B. The fistulous tract might be partially obliterated with esophageal wall mucosa
C. The bronchoscopist has failed to perform a careful and diligent inspection
D. The fistulous tract spontaneously opens and closes and can sometimes only be discovered after probing suspicious appearing areas using forceps.
E. All of the above

Q5: Which of the following best describes endobronchial abnormalities caused by sarcoidosis?

A. Mucosal nodularity, bronchial strictures, or hyperemia.
B. Mucosal edema, hypertrophy, or small raised whitish lesions.
C. Both a and b
D. Both a and b are correct, but airway abnormalities are nonspecific and can also be seen with other diseases.

Q6: A procedure is appropriately considered "nondiagnostic" when…?

A. Inspection and representative tissue samples and/or washings do not provide a diagnosis.
B. Tissue samples are obtained, but are not representative (for examples, bronchoscopic lung biopsies reveal no pathology, and contain only bronchial mucosa, but no bronchioles or alveoli).

Q7: Which of following statements about bronchoscopy-related pneumothorax (during bronchoscopic lung biopsy) is CORRECT?

A. Pneumothorax occurs more frequently when large alligator forceps are used rather than small cup forceps.
B. The overall incidence of bronchoscopy-related pneumothorax is about the same as that of percutaneous needle aspiration-related pneumothorax.
C. The reported incidence is 1-4 %.
D. Small-bore chest insertion is almost always warranted.

Q8: The inflated balloon size of a 6 Fr balloon catheter is approximately:

A. 6 mm.
B. 7 mm.
C. 10 mm.
D. 12 mm.

Q9: A transbronchial needle aspiration directed posteriorly and medially 1 cm beyond the origin of the right or left lower lobe bronchus risks entering which of the following anatomic structures?

A. The pulmonary veins.
B. The pulmonary arteries.
C. The esophagus
D. The heart

Q10: Bronchoscopic airway stents should be considered in each of the following settings EXCEPT?

A. Severe extrinsic compression of the left main bronchus in a patient with fibrosing mediastinitis, dyspnea, and cough.
B. Severe extrinsic compression of the trachea in a patient with thyroid cancer.
C. Recurrent tracheal and right main bronchial obstruction in a patient with recurrent tumor three months after laser resection.
D. Central obstruction but no known functional airways distal to the obstruction as evidenced long-standing complete atelectasis on chest radiographs and absence of ventilation on nuclear imaging studies.
E. Complex benign tracheal stricture in a patient with significant comorbidities.

The Essential Flexible Bronchoscopist©
Module VI Post-test Questions

Q1: A 74-year-old patient with subglottic tracheal stenosis and recent tracheal stent insertion (silicone stent 14 mm in diameter and 50 mm in length) presents with dyspnea and cough. A chest radiograph reveals distal migration. The patient is in severe and acute respiratory distress requiring intubation. All of the following are acceptable EXCEPT:

A. Proceed with laryngoscopic intubation using a #6 cuffless endotracheal tube
B. Proceed with bronchoscopy-assisted intubation. Select tube size dependent on airway caliber
C. Proceed with an awake bronchoscopy-assisted intubation Select tube size dependent on airway caliber.
D. Immediately paralyze the patient and proceed with laryngoscopic intubation using a #6 cuffless endotracheal tube

Q2: Which of the following statements about airway stents is FALSE?

A. In general, metal stents should be avoided in most settings of benign airway strictures.
B. Silicone stents are prone to migration and obstruction by retained secretions
C. Radiation therapy cannot be delivered because it has adverse effects on airway stents.
D. A patient with an indwelling airway stent and new symptoms such as fever, cough, or dyspnea should be rapidly evaluated for possible stent-related complications.
E. Stent-related granulation tissue formation is usually treated by laser or electrosurgical resection.

Q3: Which of the following statements about photodynamic therapy is FALSE?

A. Therapy has been FDA approved for treatment of early stage lung cancer.
B. Patients must be protected from artificial light for up to 6 weeks after treatment.
C. Tissue necrosis may cause airway obstruction and often necessitates flexible bronchoscopy for pulmonary toilet purposes.
D. Skin photosensitivity should be avoided by wearing protective clothing and eyewear for up to 6 weeks after treatment.

Q4: The esophagus usually lies:

A. Within 3 mm behind the posterior wall of the trachea and left main bronchus.
B. Directly behind the take off of the right main bronchus

C. Directly behind the trachea but anterior to the origin of the left main bronchus
D. Posterior and to the right of the distal third of the trachea.

Q5: Increased yield from transbronchial needle aspiration is most likely to result from:

A. Multiple passes and on-site examination by an expert cytopathologist.
B. Luck.
C. Applying suction while the needle is being removed from the lymph node.
D. Using the jab and thrust techniques.

Q6: Techniques of transbronchial needle aspiration are commonly referred to as all of the following, EXCEPT:

A. Jabbing method.
B. Piggy-back method
C. Cough method
D. Hub-against-the-wall method
E. Blind-insertion method

Q7: ATS nodal station 4 R is accessed by:

A. Transbronchial needle aspiration 2-4 intercartilaginous spaces posterolateral to the trachea.
B. Transbronchial needle aspiration 2-4 intercartilaginous spaces anterolateral to the trachea.
C. Transbronchial needle aspiration 2-4 intercartilaginous spaces lateral to the trachea.
D. Transbronchial needle aspiration posterolateral to the trachea at the level of the carina.

Q8: Which of the following anatomic structures lies immediately adjacent to the anterior wall of the left main bronchus and left upper lobe bronchus?

A. Left pulmonary artery
B. Aorta
C. Left pulmonary veins
D. Esophagus

Q9: Transbronchial needle aspiration of ATS station 7 is best performed by:

A. Inserting the needle in a relatively horizontal fashion against the medial wall of the right main bronchus across from and just proximal to the take-off of the right upper lobe bronchus.
B. Inserting the needle in a relatively vertical fashion against the medial wall of the right main bronchus across from and just proximal to the take-off of the right upper lobe bronchus.
C. Inserting the needle through the posterior wall of lower third of the trachea at the level of the carina.
D. Inserting the needle directly into the carina in a straight vertical direction.

Q10: All of the following are important to prevent damage to the flexible bronchoscope during transbronchial needle aspiration, EXCEPT:

A. Making certain that the needle has been withdrawn into its sheath before the sheath is withdrawn into the bronchoscope.
B. Straightening the bronchoscope before needle removal.
C. Practice.
D. Avoiding excessive flexion or extension of the tip of the bronchoscope at any time that the needle is being passed through the bronchoscope.
E. Avoid using the histology needle.

The Essential Flexible Bronchoscopist©
Answers for Post Tests Modules I – VI

ANSWERS TO MODULE I POST-TEST

1. B	2. D	3. D	4. C	5. B	6. A	7. C	8. C	9. B	10. A

ANSWERS TO MODULE II POST-TEST

1. C	2. C	3. B	4. B	5. C	6. A	7. D	8. B	9. A	10. C

ANSWERS TO MODULE III POST-TEST

1. A	2. A	3. C	4. B	5. C	6. A	7. D	8. C	9. B	10. A

ANSWERS TO MODULE IV POST-TEST

1. B	2. C	3. A	4. D	5. D	6. B	7. D	8. D	9. D	10. A

ANSWERS TO MODULE V POST-TEST

1. B	2. C	3. B	4. E	5. D	6. B	7. C	8. D	9. A	10. D

ANSWERS TO MODULE VI POST-TEST

1. A	2. C	3. B	4. A	5. A	6. E	7. B	8. C	9. A	10. E

The Essential Flexible Bronchoscopist© is found on Amazon and Kindle.

SECTION 9
Faculty Development

An Excerpt from the Train the Trainers Manual

The following section is an introduction to Bronchoscopy International's Faculty Development Program (Train the Trainers). This seminar is devoted to helping you acquire the necessary skills to teach the *Introduction to Flexible Bronchoscopy* curriculum. It is divided into two sections:

- Familiarization with the curriculum, the lectures and their administration, the models used, and the assessment tools including how they can be administered, used and scored. We refer to this basic section as the Trainer Initiation Program.
- A more in-depth discussion of the conceptual topics involved in bronchoscopy education. These topics include curriculum development, adaptation and incorporation, adult learning theory, coaching and feedback skills, individualized and group instruction, incorporation of new learning materials, assessment tools and methodologies, confidence building, audience engagement, enthusiasm generation, handling difficult learners, motivational education, and much more.

We are confident that our efforts planning and preparing this course will result in substantial learning and enjoyment on your part. We know that you will learn techniques that will assist you teaching bronchoscopy, and that you will feel increasingly comfortable incorporating many of the elements from this curriculum into your future teaching endeavors.

Because we value your assessment of our programs, we would appreciate very much having you give your attention to the evaluation forms distributed throughout this seminar. It will also be very important to complete the various self assessment and 360 degree evaluations provided, and to do your best to use a teaching portfolio documenting your teaching experiences during the course of the next year. Our instructors are always available to assist you in any way.

"Train The Trainers"

A seminar in preparation for the one-day structured program:

INTRODUCTION TO FLEXIBLE BRONCHOSCOPY

BRONCHOSCOPY INTERNATIONAL™
FOUNDATION FOR THE ADVANCEMENT OF MEDICINE
A NON-PROFIT 501 (C) 3 ORGANIZATION
(Tax ID 33-0593357, registration, San Diego, CA, USA)

"To learn, read. To know, write. To master, teach"
Hindu proverb

PURPOSE: To assure the appropriate transmission of a structured curriculum pertaining to an introductory course in flexible bronchoscopy. The purposes of such a program are to help establish a minimum standard of bronchoscopic knowledge and technical skill, initiate a more uniform approach to bronchoscopic learning, and enhance each trainer's ability to communicate and teach effectively in a style consistent with learner-centric competency-oriented and mastery training philosophies.

This structured curriculum is specifically designed to provide learners with cognitive, technical, affective, and experiential skills that are complementary to their apprenticeship-based learning in tertiary training institutions, and knowledge gained from participation in post-graduate programs sponsored by national and international medical professional associations. By participating in this faculty development seminar, participants will improve their teaching skills and be better able to incorporate all or part of the *Introduction to flexible bronchoscopy curriculum* into their own training programs and workshops.

Cost: This seminar is provided for a nominal fee as part of the many educational activities of Bronchoscopy International in partnership with national and international professional medical organizations. Programs are conducted with the official sponsorship of tertiary training institutions, and endorsement from the World Association for Bronchology and Interventional Pulmonology, and with the generous participations of equipment manufactures and simulation industry that enhance the hands-on workshops. Bronchoscopy International consists of a group of dedicated volunteer bronchoscopy experts and educators who work together because they believe that (1) knowledge should be democratized and readily accessible, and (2) patients should not suffer the burden of medical procedure-related learning.

OBJECTIVES: By the end of this seminar, the participant will be able to

1. Identify how instructors and program directors can use elements from the Bronchoscopy Education Project to document progression along the bronchoscopy learning curve from novice to competent practitioner.
2. Demonstrate how to teach the Bronchoscopy step-by-step© exercises in a lo-fidelity model using a hands-off approach to instruction.
3. Demonstrate how to teach bronchoscopic brushing and biopsy in a lo-fidelity model using a hands-off approach to instruction.
4. Demonstrate how to teach transbronchial needle aspiration in a lo-fidelity model using a hands-off approach to instruction.
5. Demonstrate how to use validated Bronchoscopy Assessment Tools© in order to objectively measure a student's technical skill.
6. Demonstrate how to use various checklists to ascertain knowledge and skill acquisition in areas relating to bronchoscopy, including informed consent, sedation, fluoroscopy, and overall competency in flexible bronchoscopy.
7. Demonstrate how to effectively create and use *Practical Approach to Bronchoscopic Decision Making*™ exercises as part of a learning curriculum.
8. Demonstrate how multiple choice questions from the Essential Flexible Bronchoscopist© can be used as part of an interactive session with learners.
9. Demonstrate the ability to incorporate interactive techniques into a didactic lecture pertaining to a structured curriculum of bronchoscopic knowledge.
10. Demonstrate the acquisition of knowledge pertaining to educational philosophies and techniques while performing open-book, problem-based learning exercises.
11. Demonstrate the ability to work as a team in order to deliver a structured curriculum of bronchoscopic knowledge.
12. Demonstrate the ability to work individually and as a team in order to provide constructive feedback about oneself and to others regarding learning skills, teaching skills, assessments, and organizational structure.

DESCRIPTION OF ACTIVITIES:

1. Before the course, participants will receive the *Introduction to Flexible Bronchoscopy* curriculum and Training Manual, as well as reading material pertaining to the philosophies and techniques of education, and selected literature pertaining to flexible bronchoscopy. These materials will be used during the seminar to acquire and improve various teaching skills.
2. Before the course, participants will become familiar with the Essential Flexible Bronchoscopist© and other components of the ever-expanding on-line curriculum. They will select two questions from the Essential Flexible Bronchoscopist© in order to practice interactive teaching during role playing exercises.

3. Each participant will contribute to the writing of a *Practical Approach* scenario, either during or prior to the seminar. This will be done as a Word document. Participants will also write a Practical Approach PowerPoint presentation using the *Practical Approach* template (templates and case examples will be provided to the participants well in advance). Working in teams, each will select a representative to present the scenario and completed exercise to the group. The group will provide constructive criticism in order to help improve the content and delivery of the PowerPoint presentation.
4. To view, review, and practice Bronchoscopy step by step© exercises. At the time of the course, each participant will perform these exercises under guidance (as if they were actually teaching them) in order to improve their teaching skills.
5. To view, review, and practice bronchoscopic brushing, biopsy, and TBNA in a lo-fidelity model. At the time of the seminar, each participant will perform these procedures under guidance (as if they were actually teaching them) in order to improve their teaching skills.
6. To repeatedly test a surrogate student in order to practice and reproduce scoring using Bronchoscopy Assessment Tools© and checklists. Scenarios will include testing of Step-by-Step exercises, specific tasks (such as going directly to the right middle lobe bronchus), and performing inspection flexible bronchoscopy, TBNA, and Brushings/biopsy in a lo-fidelity model.
7. To repeatedly test a surrogate student (role-playing exercises) using other checklists.
8. During the seminar, participants will practice working as a team in order to complete and present problem-based learning exercises, didactic lectures, interactive sessions, and 360-degree feedback.

EVALUATION: Good assessments are part of good learning and good teaching.

1. Participants will be asked to perform a self-assessment and a 360 degree assessment of their colleagues' skills and behaviors after completion of the didactic and interactive lectures.
2. Participants will be asked to perform a self-assessment and a 360 degree assessment of their colleagues' skills and behaviors after completion of the hands-on training sessions.
3. Participants will be asked to perform a self-assessment and a 360 degree assessment of their colleagues' skills and behaviors after completion of the group problem-based learning exercises.
4. At the end of the day, participants will be asked to complete a global assessment of the entire seminar, including their pre-seminar work, and to identify specific strengths and weaknesses of the seminar's curriculum and training activities.
5. During the course of one year after the seminar, participants will be asked to keep a personal portfolio of their bronchoscopy teaching activities, and to self-qualify their performance and areas of improvement.
6. During the next two years after the seminar, participants pledge to organize or participate in regional Introduction to Flexible Bronchoscopy programs in order to initiate a more uniform approach to the bronchoscopy educational process.

CERTIFICATION: After completion of this *Train the Trainers* seminar, each participant will receive a certificate of completion identifying them as a trainer for the "Introduction to flexible bronchoscopy Course" for Bronchoscopy International.

CURRICULUM FOR TRAINERS in Introduction to flexible bronchoscopy

Members of the core faculty of this curriculum are expert bronchoscopists and medical educators who have considerable experience teaching structured curricula, and who are also experienced in teaching and evaluating technical bronchoscopy skills, working one-on-one with learners, writing practical approach scenarios and presentations, creating and moderating problem-based learning sessions, as well as in facilitating or presenting interactive, simulation-based, and didactic classroom lectures. These faculty members are familiar with adult education techniques, and keep up to date with the educational process. They remain current and well read in regards to the bronchoscopy literature, and have experience working within a diverse medical cultural environment. They have been active researchers and have participated in the writing and publication of numerous peer reviewed articles, and have gained experience with the creation, validation, and use of simulation technologies.

The global purpose of this curriculum is to help create a core of expert volunteer bronchoscopists familiar with educational philosophies and techniques, and capable of designing and delivering a structured curriculum consistent with Bronchoscopy International's educational philosophies. This core group of *trainers* will be able to effectively teach students and colleagues in order to enhance cognitive knowledge, improve technical skill, and provide a forum that nurtures professionalism and competency in the context of shared decision making and ethical medical practice.

The Curriculum

Prior to attending the seminar, participants will have received a packet of materials that includes (1) the full *Introduction to flexible bronchoscopy* curriculum, (2) the Bronchoscopy Step-by-Step video exercises with commentary, (3) a set of PowerPoint Presentations with audio commentaries describing some examples of how to teach various bronchoscopic skills, and how to create a Practical Approach exercise, (4) a selection of articles pertaining to the validation and application of structured bronchoscopy curricula and simulation, (5) a selection of articles pertaining to education philosophies and techniques, (6) a selection of articles pertaining to flexible bronchoscopy techniques such as biopsy, brushings, bronchoalveolar lavage, foreign body removal, emergency intubation, endobronchial biopsy, transbronchial lung biopsy, conventional transbronchial needle aspiration, airway anatomy, history of flexible bronchoscopy, sedation, diagnostic strategies in specific diseases such as infectious lung diseases, lung cancer, and fixed and dynamic central airway obstruction, patient safety, medical ethics relating to procedures and novel technologies, and review papers pertaining to competency, professionalism, informed consent, (7) a set of bronchoscopy assessment tools and checklists, (8) a Bronchoscopy Education Project Training Manual related teaching modules, and instructional videos or their social media links.

The curriculum begins with an orientation comprised of an introductory session during which participants are oriented to the philosophy and scope of practice of Bronchoscopy International, a forum of expert volunteers dedicated to the dissemination and open acquisition of bronchoscopic knowledge. During this lecture, participants will learn more about the growing, web-based, six-part curriculum that includes: The Essential Flexible Bronchoscopist©, BronchAtlas™, Bronchoscopy Step-by-Step©, Bronchoscopy Assessment Tools©, The Art of Bronchoscopy, and Practical Approach to Bronchoscopy Decision Making©. They will learn how these instruments can be used for individual and group learning, and they will become more familiar with how they might also contribute to this on-line resource. This session will also introduce participants to some of the basic principles used in adult education, and present examples of techniques, analogies, and methods with which procedural narratives might be used to transmit message, share a technical skill, as well as rationally think through a procedural consultation.

Participants will become familiar with general vocabulary used in adult education, review pertinent articles pertaining to the use of simulation technology for training purposes, understand the complexities of competency-based training and the importance of ongoing assessments and continued learning. Participants will also become familiar with the Bronchoscopy Education Project, our attempt to initiate a more uniform, turnkey curriculum for flexible bronchoscopy training, which ultimately can be altered as needed based on regional, cultural, and institutional needs.

In summary, this introductory session will convey the major goal of the proposed curriculum, which is to create a learning environment in which participants can learn to work together as a team and have fun while teaching. In this way, future students will have a productive and joyful educational experience on their journey to attain varying degrees of competency. This will ultimately benefit patients, colleagues, and society.

Subsequent components of the curriculum are structured to elicit interest, teamwork, and individual analysis of one's knowledge and technical skill. Using a multimodality learning program, participants will experience the learning process, and thus be able to better communicate with future learners. They will experience multimedia presentations, and learn how on-site visual, auditory, and video technologies can be used to complement other educational systems. The purposes are to enhance a skill, promote knowledge, acquire experience, think through a problem-based scenario, and rationalize the decision-making process. During the course of one and a half days, activities will be divided into classroom didactic sessions, round table group discussions, individual and team presentations, and a series of hands-on technical skills training and testing using simulation-based scenarios.

We believe it is important to evaluate the process of teaching in order to improve one's own abilities. It is helpful to assess a learner's ability without judging, so that positive reinforcement can be provided. Participants will be asked to self-qualify their own learning and teaching experiences, and to provide 360-degree feedback to the other participants in their group. Questions extracted from commonly used leadership development courses were used to create specific 360-degree instruments. Although some scores may be collected by the seminar organizers for use in an ongoing research evaluation of the *Train the Trainers* Course curriculum, 360-degree assessments will always remain anonymous. Questionnaires will be tabulated and immediately returned to course participants for their personal review. During a debriefing session, faculty will be available to discuss results with the group, or later with individuals on a confidential level if desired.

One of the major strengths of this seminar is learning through shared experience within a context of facilitation. Because each seminar participant is considered an experienced bronchoscopist in his and her own right, participants should each consider themselves as "first among equals". Group exercises, however, will help participants function as a team. This is an essential element of the teaching process, because during the delivery of a structured bronchoscopy curriculum, instructors must be able to "feed off each other", providing information to learners based on experience, contradictory evidence, and opinion.

Not all practitioners think or behave alike, yet, in an effort to create a common foundation of bronchoscopic knowledge and skill, they must agree on certain principles. Many of these will be reviewed and commented upon during the seminar. In addition, participants will learn to work together in order to justify procedural decisions, approach an adult learning educational problem, appreciate the advantages and obstacles of patient-centered learning, design an introductory course curriculum, create and deliver an interactive session, and give a didactic lecture in a fixed period of time. Using a faculty panel model, participants will simulate the teaching environment of the *Introduction to flexible bronchoscopy curriculum*, and experience some of the difficulties that might be encountered when teaching this curriculum to a large group of novices or experienced bronchoscopists.

In order to help participants master some of the technical skills necessary in performing bronchoscopy step-by-step exercises, and also to share a philosophy of teaching that emphasizes guided practice rather than demonstration, several hours of the curriculum are devoted to hands-on flexible bronchoscopy training. During these sessions, participants will learn, demonstrate, and teach bronchoscopy step-by-step exercises, in addition to brushing, mucosal biopsy, and TBNA of level 4 and level 7 lymph nodes using affordable lo-fidelity airway models. If available, computer-based simulators will also be used. Participants will become familiar with validated Bronchoscopy Assessment tools, such as BSTAT and BSAT, in order to incorporate them more readily into their own training programs, or modify them according to their individual needs.

Using a hands-off approach, small groups of participants will simultaneously observe and score a course instructor learning step by step exercises. specific tasks such as going straight to the right middle love bronchus will be performed, and 10-point checklists will be used to document knowledge and skill acquisition. These tasks will be repeated as often as necessary until participants feel comfortable with the scoring process, and until a relatively high rate of inter-observer reliability is obtained. Participants will also practice specific coaching techniques such as use of positive reinforcement, correction by demonstration, correction by explanation, use of analogy, and patient-based narratives pertaining to why a specific technique may prove to be helpful when performing bronchoscopy in a real patient.

As mentioned previously, 360-degree assessments, in addition to self-qualifying assessments will be completed during the course of the program. Participants will thus be asked to self-qualify their experience and behaviors in regard to group activities, individual didactic teaching exercises, and individual hands-on teaching. They will also be asked to evaluate other participants during group activities, individual didactic teaching exercises, and during hands-on training if possible. These 360-degree assessments will be kept confidential, but are necessary to help participants learn about how they are perceived, how they perceive themselves, and to help participants modify certain behaviors, habits, manners of speech or hands-on teaching techniques. In addition, such activities help participants evaluate the process of teaching and create an environment of trust and teamwork. They also provide program organizers with feedback needed to improve the curriculum for future train-the-trainers seminars.

Overall, the seminar entails 4 hours of simulation-based hands-on training and approximately 10 hours of onsite didactics and interactive sessions, in addition to more than 10 hours of individual reading and preparation. Course work will be completed during a 1 ½ day program delivered on site at the training center, and will include a working dinner followed by a full day with snacks, lunch, coffee or tea breaks. The closing ceremony will be preceded by a summary debriefing session, and a certificate of completion will be delivered to all participants.

Table 1: Sample agenda for Train the Trainers Curriculum: Simulation-based, hands-on workshops

Program	Topic	Duration
Learning and teaching Step-by-Step	Bronchoscopy exercises**	1 hour
Standardized scoring using *Bronchoscopy Assessment Tools*	BSAT, BSTAT, BSTAT-TBLB/TBNA	1 hour
Simulation-based bronchoscopy training	Teaching TBNA using hands-off technique (instruments, patient safety, protecting the equipment, use of the assistant)	1 hour
Simulation-based module training	Informed consent, patient safety, procedural pause, sedation, fluoroscopy	1 hour

** *See Bronchoscopy Step-by-Step Poster and*

- Colt HG. Bronchoscopy Lessons. A series of lessons pertaining to aspects of bronchoscopy. (posted 2010). http://www.youtube.com/watch?v=phRv73Ik7fI&feature=related. You Tube (BronchOrg site).
- Colt HG. Bronchoscopy Education Project Rationale. http://www.youtube.com/watch?v=ogRixvyTYEA. You Tube, posted July 2010.

Table 2: Sample agenda for Train the Trainers Curriculum: Didactic/Interactive Sessions and Roundtable Discussions

Program	Topics	Duration
Orientation	Introduction to the curriculum, learning philosophies, and methods	1 hour
Interactive session using the Essential Bronchoscopist	Each participant uses one or two questions from the EB to address the audience and teach about a topic	1 hour
Problem-based learning group exercise followed by debriefing	Educational philosophies using 10-point checklists and assessment tools and incorporating them into a training program	1.5 hours
Didactic lecture	In groups of two or three, participants deliver one of the *Introduction to flexible bronchoscopy* curriculum presentations	1 hour
Interactive session using audience participation system or true/false exercises	In groups of two or three, participants generate controversy and consensus regarding specific bronchoscopic strategies and results	1 hour
Practical Approach Exercise	In groups of four, an individual PA scenario and exercise is created using the PA PowerPoint template and the four-box approach to procedural decision making	30 minutes-one hour
Practical Approach didactic lecture	An individual from each group delivers the presentation in 10-15 minutes	30 minutes-one hour
Problem-based learning group exercise and debriefing	Educational techniques and structure: designing a one- or two-day curriculum (goals, content, obstacles, results)	1.5 hours
Improving performance (didactic lecture)	How to become an effective trainer	30 minutes
360-degree feedback and self-qualified assessments	Based on behavior and performance during group exercises, and individual teaching assignment	30 minutes

Working dinner Sample agenda

- Welcome-Icebreaker
- Introductions
- Program objectives
- Educational philosophies
- Group and individual assignments: begin group assignments

SECTION 10

Checklists

A collection of checklists and user instructions:

- Moderate sedation
- Fluoroscopy
- Informed consent
- Procedural pause and Patient safety
- Practical Approach
- Bronchoscopy step-by-step
- Proctored bronchoscopy
- IFB Program completion

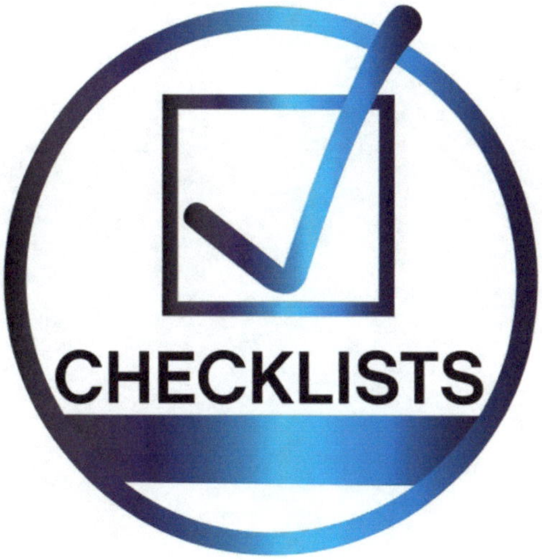

Scoring Recommendations for CHECKLISTS

(Informed Consent, Procedural Pause, Fluoroscopy, Moderate Sedation, Patient Safety, Proctored Bronchoscopy,)

The goal of these checklists is to monitor a learner's progress from *novice* (Score < 60) to *advanced beginner* (Score 60-79), *intermediate* (score 80-99), and *competent* (score 100). The instructor should ascertain, by observing the learner's performance that each of the TEN elements in each checklist are covered satisfactorily. The frequency with which these checklists are used is at the discretion of program organizers.

Repeated testing demonstrates progressive knowledge and skill acquisition as learners climb the learning curve. When there is more one entry in an item category, partial scores for each entry are possible to help identify areas requiring additional training (for example, if there are two entries under one item, and a score of 10 is required for the item, each entry may be scored 5 points). Using mastery training philosophy, competency is the minimum acceptable standard. We therefore recommend that the maximum score possible be attained for each item to be scored as satisfactory, and that 100% scores for all items be necessary for the bronchoscopist to be considered to have satisfactorily satisfied training requirements measured using the checklist.

To maximize objective scoring, each task has been defined explicitly. Participation in *Train-the-Trainers* programs is encouraged to assist instructors achieve interobserver reliability, and to use this program to its fullest potential.

Scores can be plotted on a graph, and programs may choose their own cut-offs for a PASS grade. We recommend that a PASS grade warrants a score of 100.

In the absence of studies demonstrating standard normograms as is done for high-stakes testing, consensus of world renowned experts was obtained to delineate cut-off scores for the following four categories.

Category	Score
Novice	< 60
Advanced Beginner	60-79
Intermediate	80-99
Competent	100

Specific instructions are marked by an asterisk (*).

MODERATE SEDATION 10-Point CHECKLIST*

Learner ______________________________ Training Year ______________

Faculty ______________________________ Date ____________________

☐ Interactive session ☐ Patient environment

Educational Item* Items 1-10 scored 10 points each. (Partial points are possible)	**Satisfactory Yes/No**
1. Definitions ☐ Moderate sedation ☐ Deep sedation	Yes / No
2. Able to obtain moderate sedation informed consent	Yes / No
3. Able to describe ASA classification ☐ 1 ☐ 2 ☐ 3 ☐ 4 ☐ 5	Yes / No
4. Able to identify high risk patients	Yes / No
5. Able to describe potential contraindications	Yes / No
6. Able to list equipment that must be available	Yes / No
7. Sedation agents: role, dosage, precautions ☐ Midazolam ☐ Fentanyl	Yes / No
8. Reversal agents: role, dosage, precautions ☐ Flumazenil ☐ Naloxone	Yes / No
9. Able to describe how to respond to complications such as ☐ Vomiting ☐ Seizure	Yes / No
10A. Able to describe how to respond to over-sedation and ☐ Hypotension ☐ Airway obstruction	Yes / No
10B. Able to describe how to respond to over-sedation and ☐ Hypoxemia ☐ Respiratory failure	Yes / No

* Contains elements required by ACGME (patient care, medical knowledge, practice-based learning and improvement, interpersonal communication skills, professionalism, and systems-based practice).

FINAL GRADE PASS FAIL **SCORE** _______/100

USER INSTRUCTIONS

Moderate Sedation Checklist

Questions pertaining to sedation can be asked during a separate simulation session or during a patient encounter. The learner will have received the sedation synopsis as well as any institution-specific guidelines and protocols. A passing score of 100, although somewhat subjective, is encouraged.

Educational Item* Items 1-10 scored 10 points each (partial points are possible)	**Satisfactory Yes/No**
1. Definitions ☐ Moderate sedation ☐ Deep sedation	Yes / No
2. Able to obtain moderate sedation informed consent	Yes / No
3. Able to describe ASA classification ☐ 1 ☐ 2 ☐ 3 ☐ 4 ☐ 5	Yes / No
4. Able to identify high risk patients	Yes / No
5. Able to describe potential contraindications	Yes / No
6. Able to list equipment that must be available	Yes / No
7. Sedation agents: role, dosage, precautions ☐ Midazolam ☐ Fentanyl	Yes / No
8. Reversal agents: role, dosage, precautions ☐ Flumazenil ☐ Naloxone	Yes / No
9. Able to describe how to respond to complications such as ☐ Vomiting ☐ Seizure	Yes / No
10A. Able to describe how to respond to over-sedation and ☐ Hypotension ☐ Airway obstruction	Yes / No
10B. Able to describe how to respond to over-sedation and ☐ Hypoxemia ☐ Respiratory failure	Yes / No

* Contains elements required by ACGME (patient care, medical knowledge, practice-based learning and improvement, interpersonal communication skills, professionalism, and systems- based practice).

FINAL GRADE PASS FAIL **SCORE** ______/100

FLUOROSCOPY 10-Point CHECKLIST*

Learner ______________________________ Training Year _____________

Faculty ______________________________ Date ____________________

☐ Interactive session ☐ Patient environment

Educational Item* Items 1-10 scored 10 points each (partial points are possible)	**Satisfactory Yes/No**
1. Able to list indications for using fluoroscopy	Yes / No
2. Able to describe the relevance of voltage and amperage ☐ For image quality ☐ For patient safety	Yes / No
3. Able to describe consequences of resolution, distortion, and lag ☐ For image quality ☐ For patient safety	Yes / No
4. Able to describe consequences of brightness and contrast ☐ For image quality ☐ For patient safety	Yes / No
5. Able to describe dangers of scattered radiation	Yes / No
6. Able to describe techniques to improve visibility of fluoroscopic image	Yes / No
7. Able to describe techniques used to reduce patient radiation exposure	Yes / No
8. Able to describe techniques used to reduce operator radiation exposure	Yes / No
9. Able to describe special precautions in case of suspected or known pregnancy ☐ Patients ☐ Health care providers	Yes / No
10. Able to describe basic operation procedures	Yes / No

* Contains elements required by ACGME (patient care, medical knowledge, practice-based learning and improvement, interpersonal communication skills, professionalism, and systems-based practice).

FINAL GRADE PASS FAIL **SCORE** _______/100

USER INSTRUCTIONS

Fluoroscopy Checklist

Questions pertaining to fluoroscopy can be asked during a separate simulation session or during a patient encounter. The learner will have received the fluoroscopy synopsis as well as any institution-specific guidelines and protocols. A passing score of 100, although somewhat subjective, is encouraged.

Educational Item* Items 1-10 scored 10 points each (partial points are possible)	**Satisfactory Yes/No**
1. Able to list indications for using fluoroscopy	Yes / No
2. Able to describe the relevance of voltage and amperage ☐ For image quality ☐ For patient safety	Yes / No
3. Able to describe consequences of resolution, distortion, and lag ☐ For image quality ☐ For patient safety	Yes / No
4. Able to describe consequences of brightness and contrast ☐ For image quality ☐ For patient safety	Yes / No
5. Able to describe dangers of scattered radiation	Yes / No
6. Able to describe techniques to improve visibility of fluoroscopic image	Yes / No
7. Able to describe techniques used to reduce patient radiation exposure	Yes / No
8. Able to describe techniques used to reduce operator radiation exposure	Yes / No
9. Able to describe special precautions in case of suspected or known pregnancy ☐ Patients ☐ Health care providers	Yes / No
10. Able to describe basic operation procedures	Yes / No

* Contains elements required by ACGME (patient care, medical knowledge, practice-based learning and improvement, interpersonal communication skills, professionalism, and systems-based practice).

FINAL GRADE PASS FAIL **SCORE** _______/100

INFORMED CONSENT 10-Point CHECKLIST*

Learner ______________________ Training Year ____________

Faculty ______________________ Date ________________

☐ Simulation Bronchoscopy Workshop ☐ Patient-based Bronchoscopy Scenario

Educational Item* Items 1-10 scored 10 points each (Partial points are possible)	**Satisfactory Yes/No**
1. Able to define "Informed Consent": ☐ Informed decision-making regarding indications and expected outcomes, ☐ Conflict of interest ☐ Protection from liability ☐ Provides opportunity to assess management strategies ☐ Provides opportunity to discuss risks, benefits, and alternatives	Yes / No
2. Able to discuss diagnosis and pertinent clinical issues	Yes / No
3. Able to describe the purpose of the procedure	Yes / No
4. Able to describe the nature of the procedure	Yes / No
5. Able to describe procedure-related risks	Yes / No
6. Able to describe procedure-related benefits	Yes / No
7. Able to describe alternative procedures regardless of cost or health care coverage	Yes / No
8. Able to describe potential risks and benefits from choosing the alternatives	Yes / No
9. Able to describe the risks and benefits of not performing the procedure or not choosing any of the alternatives	Yes / No
10. Able to demonstrate "effectiveness" of the informed consent process by asking the patient to explain in his or her own words, their understanding of the procedure	Yes / No

* Contains elements required by ACGME (patient care, medical knowledge, practice-based learning and improvement, interpersonal communication skills, professionalism, and systems-based practice).

FINAL GRADE PASS FAIL **SCORE** ______/100

USER INSTRUCTIONS

Informed consent Checklist

Educational Item* Items 1-10 scored 10 points each (Partial points are possible)
1. Able to define "Informed Consent" ☐ Informed decision-making regarding indications and expected outcomes, ☐ conflict of interest ☐ Protection from liability ☐ Provides opportunity to assess management strategies ☐ Provides opportunity to discuss risks, benefits, and alternatives * The instructor may wish that the student be able to address some of the history of informed consent, and explain how and why informed consent plays a prominent role in medicine today.
2. Able to discuss diagnosis and pertinent clinical issues * Which diagnostic elements and clinical information help guide a patient's choice of procedures? Why is this particular procedure being performed based on diagnosis and clinical issues? This provides the background to the informed consent process and opens the door for a dialogue with the patient so that the patient understands that simple authorization to perform the procedures is not what is being requested.
3. Able to describe the purpose of the procedure * Based on the clinical picture, the procedure is placed into context and the different elements of the procedure (such as to obtain lung tissue, or to obtain lung secretions to look at under the microscope in order to detect infection) are described.
4. Able to describe the nature of the procedure * The procedure is described in layman's terms.
5. Able to describe procedure-related risks * Risks applicable to the procedure are noted; the student may offer a few questions and answers, such as when can the patient eat, will the procedure hurt, is there a chance for bleeding or lung collapse. Some patients may fear death, and so this also may need to be addressed. A description of risks can increase both state and trait anxiety, and therefore, patients should probably be asked about their anxiety level and whether medication or other interventions (music, hand-holding, family members present at bedside, etc) are desired.
6. Able to describe procedure-related benefits * Benefits should be described clearly, such as early diagnosis leads to early treatment, may avoid need for more invasive tests, ability to remove patients from isolation, provide information to other doctors to assist with therapeutic and diagnostic strategies, certain illnesses might be excluded so as to simplify further work-up.

7. Able to describe alternative procedures regardless of cost or health care coverage * Alternatives to bronchoscopy should be cited and described; these might include, for example, invasive procedures such as open surgery, mediastinoscopy, percutaneous needle aspiration, and noninvasive procedures such as radiographic studies, etc.
8. Able to describe potential risks and benefits from choosing the alternatives * The risks and benefits from each of the alternatives should be addressed and explained. They can be compared to those of bronchoscopy, and the physician can provide expert opinion as to why bronchoscopy is being proposed and recommended.
9. Able to describe the risks and benefits of not performing the procedure or not choosing any of the alternatives * If bronchoscopy is not performed, the patient should be told about potential consequences, whether or not alternatives are chosen, such as, for example, delayed diagnosis, prolonged illness, endangerment, need for different modes of surveillance or subsequent diagnostic tests or therapeutic measures.
10. Able to demonstrate "effectiveness" of the informed consent process by asking the patient to explain in his or her own words, their understanding of the procedure * The patient should be asked to describe the bronchoscopy and its consequences in general terms. This also provides an opportunity for dialogue.

* Contains elements required by ACGME (patient care, medical knowledge, practice-based learning and Improvement, interpersonal communication skills, professionalism, and systems-based practice).

FINAL GRADE PASS FAIL **SCORE** _______/100

PROCEDURAL PAUSE and PATIENT SAFETY 10-Point CHECKLIST*

Learner ______________________________ Training Year _____________

Faculty ______________________________ Date ____________________

☐ Simulation Bronchoscopy Workshop ☐ Patient-based Bronchoscopy Scenario

Educational Item* Items 1-10 scored 10 points each (Partial points are possible)	**Satisfactory Yes/No**
1. Able to define "Procedural Pause" as: ☐ Time-Out ☐ Wrong patient, site, procedure ☐ Team communication/patient understanding ☐ Mandatory in USA	Yes / No
2. Able to describe requirements of the procedural pause: ☐ Immediately before procedure ☐ Correct site, position, procedure ☐ Correct patient ☐ Pertinent medical records and equipment ☐ Verbal acknowledgements by all team members ☐ Elimination of environmental distractions	Yes / No
3. Able to describe the team leader's role	Yes / No
4. Able to describe the nursing team's role	Yes / N0
5. Able to describe the patient's role	Yes / N0
6. Able to describe other person's roles (technicians, other physicians)	Yes / No
7. Able to list the elements that must be covered: ☐ Patient ☐ Procedure ☐ Side and site ☐ Informed consent ☐ Medical records and equipment ☐ Medications ☐ Allergies/drug reactions ☐ Safety concerns based on history	Yes / No
8. Able to address behaviors in case of distractions	Yes / No
9. Able to describe behaviors in case of disagreements	Yes / No
10. Able to describe other elements that help assure a culture of safety: ☐ Communication ☐ Ability to prevent complications ☐ Ability to respond to complications ☐ Universal precautions ☐ Droplet, and Airborne pathogen precautions	Yes / No

* Contains elements required by ACGME (patient care, medical knowledge, practice-based learning and improvement, interpersonal communication skills, professionalism, and systems-based practice).

FINAL GRADE PASS FAIL **SCORE** _______/100

USER INSTRUCTIONS

Procedural Pause and Patient Safety Checklist

1. Able to define "Procedural Pause" as ☐ Time Out ☐ Wrong patient, site, procedure ☐ Team communication/patient understanding ☐ Mandatory in USA
2. Able to describe requirements of the procedural pause ☐ Immediately before procedure ☐ Correct site, position, procedure ☐ Correct patient ☐ Pertinent medical records and equipment ☐ Verbal acknowledgements by all team members ☐ Elimination of environmental distractions
3. Able to describe the team leader's role * Mark the site if applicable, state name, patient, and procedure being performed, lead the time out, assure that all distractions are avoided during the time, requests a new time-out in case distractions occur, assures that time-out is being done according to protocol, addresses discrepancies, cancels procedure if all elements are not ascertained, modifies procedural strategy if applicable according to results of the time out.
4. Able to describe the nursing team's role * Assures patient identification using at least two independent identifiers, assures right side right patient, right procedure, reviews and reads informed consent, assures appropriate medical records and equipment are available, assures appropriate response to complications or adverse events is possible.
5. Able to describe the patient's role * If alert, able to state name, agree with procedure and site, signal family members who might be present.
6. Able to describe other person's roles (technicians other physicians) * Able to state name and role.
7. Able to list the elements that must be covered ☐ Patient ☐ Procedure ☐ Side and site ☐ Informed consent ☐ Medical records and equipment ☐ Medications ☐ Allergies/drug reactions ☐ Safety concerns based on history
8. Able to address behaviors in case of distractions * No one should enter or leave the room during the time-out; any interruptions should prompt renewing the time-out; if a new or second procedure is being performed, time-out should be repeated; individuals should remain silent so that all present can focus on the time-out being performed.

9. Able to describe behaviors in case of disagreements * Verbal comments, behavior modification during or after the time-out; anyone should be able to disagree with what is being said during the time-out if it is inconsistent with the informed consent, predesignated procedural strategy, or clinical suspicions.
10. Able to describe other elements that help assure a culture of safety: ☐ Communication ☐ Ability to prevent complications ☐ Ability to respond to complications ☐ Universal precautions ☐ Droplet, and Airborne pathogen precautions

* It is understood that differences between institutions and countries exist. Guidelines specific to each institution/country of practice are provided. General rules and concepts, are covered in the simulation session.

PRACTICAL APPROACH 10 Point CHECKLIST*

Learner ______________________ Training Year ______________

Faculty ______________________ Date ______________

☐ Instructor-learner 30 minute session ☐ Daily rounds & bronchoscopy consultation

Educational Item* Items 1-10 scored 10 points each (Partial points are possible)	**Satisfactory Yes/No**
1. Initial evaluation A ☐ Physical examination, laboratory tests, and functional assessment ☐ Comorbidities	Yes / No
2. Initial evaluation B ☐ Support system ☐ Preferences and expectations	Yes / No
3. Procedural strategies A ☐ Indications, contraindications, expected results ☐ Operator and team experience and expertise	Yes / No
4. Procedural strategies B ☐ Risk-benefits and therapeutic alternatives ☐ Informed consent	Yes / No
5. Techniques and results A ☐ Anesthesia and perioperative care ☐ Techniques and instruments	Yes / No
6. Techniques and results B ☐ Anatomic dangers and other risks ☐ Results and complications	Yes / No
7. Long-term management plan A ☐ Outcome assessment ☐ Follow-up tests and procedures	Yes / No
8. Long-term management plan B ☐ Referrals to other specialists ☐ Quality improvement and team evaluation	Yes / No
9. Able to answer case-specific questions ☐ Question 1 ☐ Question 2 ☐ Question 3	Yes / No
10. General ability to provide evidence for and rationally justify decision making ☐ Subjective assessment of learner ability	Yes / No

* Contains elements required by ACGME (patient care, medical knowledge, practice-based learning and improvement, interpersonal communication skills, professionalism, and systems-based practice).

FINAL GRADE PASS FAIL **SCORE** ______/100

USER INSTRUCTIONS

Practical Approach Checklist

This practical approach exercise is held as a 30-minute session between learner and instructor, similar to an "oral examination". Of course, programs including Practical Approach-like discussions for each bronchoscopy consultation may choose to forego a formal session. Using a structured format (the four boxes), learners and instructors are more certain to cover in as great a depth as desired all aspects of a procedure: strategy and planning, techniques and instruments, and response to complications. Because each element is important, items are equally weighted at ten points each with no partial points given. A passing score of 100, although somewhat subjective, is encouraged.

Educational Item* Items 1-10 scored 10 points each (Partial points are possible)	**Satisfactory Yes/No**
1. Initial evaluation A ☐ Physical examination, laboratory tests, and functional assessment ☐ Comorbidities	Yes / No
2. Initial evaluation B ☐ Support system ☐ Preferences and expectations	Yes / No
3. Procedural strategies A ☐ Indications, contraindications, expected results ☐ Operator and team experience and expertise	Yes / No
4. Procedural strategies B ☐ Risk-benefits and therapeutic alternatives ☐ Informed consent	Yes / No
5. Techniques and results A ☐ Anesthesia and perioperative care ☐ Techniques and instruments	Yes / No
6. Techniques and results B ☐ Anatomic dangers and other risks ☐ Results and complications	Yes / No
7. Long-term management plan A ☐ Outcome assessment ☐ Follow-up tests and procedures	Yes / No
8. Long-term management plan B ☐ Referrals to other specialists ☐ Quality improvement and team evaluation	Yes / No
9. Able to answer case-specific questions ☐ Question 1 ☐ Question 2 ☐ Question 3	Yes / No
10. General ability to provide evidence for and rationally justify decision making ☐ Subjective assessment of learner ability	Yes / No

* Contains elements required by ACGME (patient care, medical knowledge, practice-based learning and improvement, interpersonal communication skills, professionalism, and systems-based practice).

FINAL GRADE PASS FAIL **SCORE** ______/100

BRONCHOSCOPY STEP BY STEP© 10 point CHECKLIST

Learner ______________________________ Training Year ______________

Faculty ______________________________ Date ____________________

☐ Simulation session ☐ Patient environment

Educational Items Each item 1-10 valued at 10 points (No partial scores unless where indicated)	**Satisfactory Yes/No**
1. **Step 1** Nose to larynx (if not applicable, score as satisfactory) ☐ Atraumatic, gentle ☐ Correct path, larynx easily visualized	Yes / No
2. **Step 2** Larynx to subglottis ☐ Scope kept midline ☐ Able to pass cords atraumatically	Yes / No
3. **Step 3** Follow the curve to the carina ☐ Scope kept midline, well controlled, no airway wall trauma	Yes / No
4. **Step 4** Carina to Right, Carina to Left, Carina Right/Left/Neutral ☐ Carina-R ☐ Carina- L ☐ R – L- Neutral	Yes / No
5. **Step 5** Down/up Left bronchus—Down/up Right bronchus ☐ Down the L (5 points) ☐ Down the R (5 points)	Yes / No
6. **Step 6** Main Bronchus to Lobar bronchi (2 points each lobe) ☐ LMB to LUL ☐ LMB to LLL ☐ RMB to RUL ☐ RMB to BI ☐ RMB to RLL	Yes / No
7. **Step 7L** Left segmental anatomy except for basal pyramid (2 points each segmental series) ☐ LB1+2 ☐ LB 3 ☐ LB 4-5-6 ☐ LB7 (if present) ☐ entrance to LLL basal segments	Yes / No
8. **Step 7R** Right segmental anatomy except for basal pyramid (2 points each segmental series) ☐ RB1 ☐ RB2 ☐ RB3 ☐ RB 4-5-6 ☐ entrance to RB7 and RLL basal segments	Yes / No
9. **Step 8L** Left lower lobe basal segments ☐ LB 8-9-10 (pan pan pan)	Yes / No
10. **Step 8R** Right lower lobe basal segments ☐ RB 7- 8 – 9 -10 (DÁrtagnan and the 3 musketeers)	Yes / No

* A score of 100 percent is warranted to PASS. Items 1-10 for which partial points are obtained should be scored as NO. Partial points are designed to identify learning needs.

FINAL GRADE PASS FAIL **SCORE** _______/100

USER INSTRUCTIONS

Bronchoscopy Step by Step© Checklist

Learners are asked to perform each exercise in or out of sequence. Ideally exercises can be learned in sequence, and then put together in groups of exercise until a complete bronchoscopic inspection is performed. Attention is paid to posture, hand positions, body positions, and diligence in respecting the following principles: Decision/Intention/Control, and Economy of movement. The bronchoscope is kept in the midline as much as possible. The Bronchoscopy step by step© instructional video is shown during hands-on sessions.

Educational Items Each item 1-10 valued at 10 points (No partial scores unless where indicated)	**Satisfactory Yes/No**
1. **Step 1** Nose to larynx (if not applicable, score as satisfactory) ☐ Atraumatic, gentle ☐ Correct path, larynx easily visualized	Yes / No
2. **Step 2** Larynx to subglottis ☐ Scope kept midline ☐ Able to pass cords atraumatically	Yes / No
3. **Step 3** Follow the curve to the carina ☐ Scope kept midline, well controlled, no airway wall trauma	Yes / No
4. **Step 4** Carina to Right, Carina to Left, Carina Right/Left/Neutral ☐ Carina-R ☐ Carina- L ☐ R – L- Neutral	Yes / No
5. **Step 5** Down/up Left bronchus—Down/up Right bronchus ☐ Down the L (5 points) ☐ Down the R (5 points)	Yes / No
6. **Step 6** Main Bronchus to Lobar bronchi (2 points each lobe) ☐ LMB to LUL ☐ LMB to LLL ☐ RMB to RUL ☐ RMB to BI ☐ RMB to RLL	Yes / No
7. **Step 7L** Left segmental anatomy except for basal pyramid (2 points each segmental series) ☐ LB1+2 ☐ LB 3 ☐ LB 4-5-6 ☐ LB7 (if present) ☐ entrance to LLL basal segments	Yes / No
8. **Step 7R** Right segmental anatomy except for basal pyramid (2 points each segmental series) ☐ RB1 ☐ RB2 ☐ RB3 ☐ RB 4-5-6 ☐ entrance to RB7 and RLL basal segments	Yes / No
9. **Step 8L** Left lower lobe basal segments ☐ LB 8-9-10 (pan pan pan)	Yes / No
10. **Step 8R** Right lower lobe basal segments ☐ RB 7- 8 – 9 -10 (DÁrtagnan and the 3 musketeers)	Yes / No

* A score of 100 percent is warranted to PASS. Items 1-10 for which partial points are obtained should be scored as NO. Partial points are only designed to identify learning needs.

FINAL GRADE PASS FAIL **SCORE** _______/100

PROCTORED FLEXIBLE BRONCHOSCOPY 10-Point CHECKLIST*

Learner ______________________________ Training Year ______________

Faculty ______________________________ Date ______________________

☐ Simulation Bronchoscopy Workshop ☐ Patient-based Bronchoscopy Scenario

Educational Item* Items 1-10 scored 10 points each (Partial points are possible)	**Satisfactory Yes/No**
1. Formulation of effective plan and strategy: ☐ Informed consent obtained, signed and in medical record ☐ History and physical ☐ Review imaging studies ☐ Cost-effective practice ☐ Use of information resources ☐ Applies evidence-based medicine ☐ Use of systems resources	Yes / No
2. Patient safety: ☐ ASA assessment ☐ Airway assessment ☐ Allergies ☐ Medications ☐ Comorbidities	Yes / No
3. Patient safety: ☐ Positioning ☐ Supplemental oxygen ☐ Vital signs ☐ Suction ☐ Bite-block and/or ET tube if applicable ☐ Verifies ability to respond to complications and accessibility of resuscitation equipment	Yes / No
4. Patient and procedural team safety: ☐ Protection from radiation/lead shielding; badge use ☐ Eye protection ☐ Knowledgeable use of fluoroscopy ☐ Hand disinfection ☐ Universal precautions ☐ Time-Out.	Yes / No
5. Procedure: ☐ Premedication ☐ Moderate sedation ☐ Topical anesthetic	Yes / No
6. Procedure: ☐ Scope insertion ☐ Topical anesthetic ☐ Passage through vocal cords ☐ Empathy and communication with patient	Yes / No
7. Procedure: ☐ Inspection of tracheobronchial tree ☐ Identification of abnormalities ☐ Atraumatic removal of bronchoscope	Yes / No
8. Procedure: ☐ BAL ☐ Mucosal biopsy ☐ Lung biopsy ☐ Brush ☐ TBNA ☐ EBUS	Yes / No
9. Communication with staff, patient, and patient family ☐ Puts needs of patient first ☐ Punctuality ☐ Respect ☐ Listening skills ☐ Personal appearance ☐ Initiative & Motivation ☐ Empathy ☐ Honesty ☐ Accepts responsibility	Yes / No
10. Documentation/procedure note ☐ Informative ☐ Accurate ☐ Communication with colleagues	Yes / No

* Contains elements required by ACGME (patient care, medical knowledge, practice-based learning and improvement, interpersonal communication skills, professionalism, and systems-based practice).

FINAL GRADE PASS FAIL **SCORE** _______/100

USER INSTRUCTIONS

Proctored Flexible Bronchoscopy Checklist

Educational Item*   Items 1-10 scored 10 points (partial points are possible)
1. Formulation of effective plan and strategy   ☐ Informed consent obtained, signed and in medical record   ☐ Review imaging studies   ☐ Use of information resources   ☐ Use of systems resources   ☐ History and physical   ☐ Cost-effective practice   ☐ Applies evidence-based medicine   * The instructor should be certain that the student has obtained the informed consent and that it is signed and in the chart. The student should be able to describe pertinent clinical and radiographic findings and to use evidence-based medicine in addition to any other information gained from other resources, such as faculty expert opinion, advice, and requests by referring physicians, to justify the procedure being performed. The student should be able to describe the use of institutional resources, and use them according to institutional practices, such as fluoroscopy, ultrasound, computed tomography, electrocautery and other instruments and equipment. This also includes nursing surveillance, respiratory therapy assistance, need for procedure suite, operating theater or intensive care unit. Cost-effectiveness can be discussed in regards to other diagnostic or therapeutic modalities, but also how bronchoscopy may or may not increase or decrease health-related expenditures in the context of the patient's diagnosis and treatment plan.
2. Patient safety: ☐ ASA assessment ☐ Airway assessment ☐ Allergies ☐ Medications ☐ Comorbidities   * ASA and Airway assessments should be performed according to the institution's guidelines. Allergies, medications, especially anticoagulants and antiplatelet agents should be noted, comorbidities that might increase the risk of adverse events should also be described and identified.
3. Patient safety: ☐ Positioning   ☐ Supplemental oxygen   ☐ Vital signs   ☐ Suction   ☐ Bite-block and/or ET tube if applicable   ☐ Verifies ability to respond to complications and accessibility of resuscitation equipment   * These measures should be taken according to institutional biases and protocols.

4. Patient and procedural team safety: ☐ Protection from radiation/lead shielding, badge use ☐ Eye protection ☐ Knowledgeable use of fluoroscopy ☐ Hand disinfection ☐ Universal precautions ☐ Time-Out. * Students should be observed as they comply with these safety measures. Additional information pertaining to time-out, universal precautions, and knowledge of fluoroscopy are provided in the modules. Protocols may vary among institutions.
5. Procedure: ☐ Premedication ☐ Moderate sedation ☐ Topical anesthetic * These should be administered according to institutional biases and according to protocols.
6. Procedure: ☐ Scope insertion ☐ Topical anesthetic ☐ Passage through vocal cords ☐ Empathy and communication with patient * Done according to institutional practices. Empathy and communication with the patient should be observed. Students should be able to speak comfortably and reassuringly with their patient. Open dialogues should be encouraged to enhance confidence and decrease patient anxiety.
7. Procedure: ☐ Inspection of tracheobronchial tree ☐ Identification of abnormalities ☐ Atraumatic removal of bronchoscope * Performed according to institutional practices.
8. Procedure: ☐ BAL ☐ Mucosal biopsy ☐ Lung biopsy ☐ Brush ☐ TBNA ☐ EBUS * Performed according to institutional practices. It is recognized that not all patients will undergo all of these procedures, therefore, if the institution desires, a different proctored checklist can be completed for each (or each set) of the procedures listed.
9. Communication with staff, patient, and patient family ☐ Puts needs of patient first ☐ Punctuality ☐ Respect ☐ Listening skills ☐ Personal appearance ☐ Initiative & Motivation ☐ Empathy ☐ Honesty ☐ Accepts responsibility * These are for the most part subjective assessments, and also require feedback from nursing staff. Students should be told that they will be judged on these items during the course of their training, so that they can obtain feedback from their instructors and improve their performance in these areas.
10. Documentation/procedure note ☐ Informative ☐ Accurate ☐ Communication with colleagues * Procedure notes may vary according to institution; however, in general, the note should be informative, telling a story about the procedure that referring physicians can understand. The note should be accurate regarding what was done, why it was done, and how it was done. Procedure-related adverse events should be described. Communication with colleagues should be observed, by watching how the student interacts with the nursing team, other physicians, and with referring physicians. While this element is also, for the most part subjective, in general, communication should be informative, accurate polite, and considerate.

* Contains elements required by ACGME (patient care, medical knowledge, practice-based learning and improvement, interpersonal communication skills, professionalism, and systems-based practice).

FINAL GRADE PASS FAIL **SCORE** _______/100

Recommendations for Using the Introduction to Flexible Bronchoscopy Program Completion Checklist

This checklist contains all of the elements comprised in the Introduction to flexible bronchoscopy program curriculum. The purpose of this curriculum is to help trainees climb the learning curve from novice and advanced beginner to intermediate and then competent bronchoscopist able to perform flexible bronchoscopy independently. Not all learners will progress at the same speed[1]. It is also assumed that learners may become competent at certain procedures before they become competent in others. The frequency with which the checklists and assessments tools pertaining to the individual components of the curriculum are administered is based on user discretion.

This curriculum assures that all learners have completed certain materials to the satisfaction of their instructors. It is understood that some may need to repeat certain elements of the curriculum until they obtain a passing grade. Some institutions may wish for their trainees to repeat parts of the curriculum during the course of their training (yearly for example, or during the months prior to completing their training). To maximize objective scoring, each element in the program checklist has been defined explicitly. Participation in *Train-the-Trainers* programs is encouraged to help instructors achieve inter-relater reliability and use this program to its fullest potential.

A PASS grade signifies that each student has achieved a satisfactory (passing) score in each of the ten elements contained in the curriculum. The overall number of procedures performed by the student should also be recorded. We recommend that learners keep a diary-log of their procedures, and that program directors conduct feedback sessions with students to monitor patient-care related outcomes.

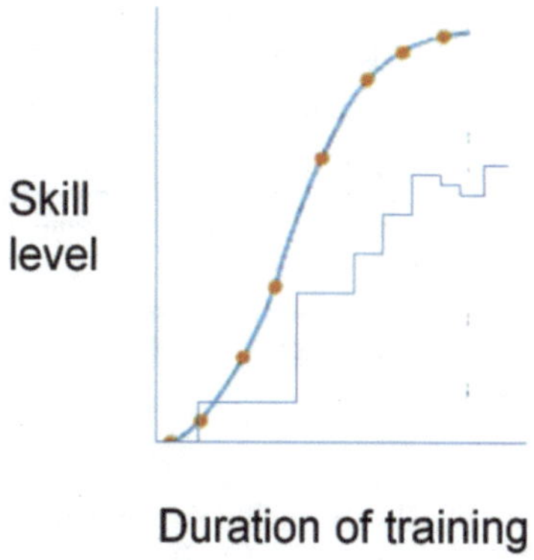

[1] German psychologist Hermann Ebbinghaus (1850-1909) is credited with originally describing the learning curve in his work on memory (see RH Wozniak. Introduction to Memory. Classics in psychology 1855-1914: Historical essays. Bristol UK, Thoemmes Press, 1999). Learning curves can be mathematically calculated and may have different shapes representing incremental change, including a series of plateaus, rises and dips, and the traditional ogive "S" shaped curve.

Introduction to Flexible Bronchoscopy Program Program Completion Checklist

Educational Item*	Completed Yes/No	Assessment Item	Pass/Fail/Incomplete
1. Participation in regional introductory course	Yes / No	Post-test scores Target 12/20 (60% correct) Score _______%	Pass / Fail / Incomplete
2. Assigned reading: *The Essential Bronchoscopist*	Yes / No	Post-test scores Target 7/10 (70% correct)	Pass / Fail / Incomplete
Module 1	Yes / No	Score _______	Pass / Fail / Incomplete
Module 2	Yes / No	Score _______	Pass / Fail / Incomplete
Module 3	Yes / No	Score _______	Pass / Fail / Incomplete
Module 4	Yes / No	Score _______	Pass / Fail / Incomplete
Module 5	Yes / No	Score _______	Pass / Fail / Incomplete
Module 6	Yes / No	Score _______	Pass / Fail / Incomplete
3. *Sedation module*	Yes/No	Score _______	Pass / Fail / Incomplete
4. *Fluoroscopy Module*	Yes/No	Score _______	Pass / Fail / Incomplete
5. Informed consent, patient safety, and procedural pause simulation workshops	Yes / No Yes / No Yes / No	IC 10-pt Checklist Target 100% Score ______% on each	Pass / Fail / Incomplete
6. Informed consent, patient safety, and procedural pause patient-based scenarios	Yes / No Yes / No Yes / No	IC 10-pt Checklist Target 100% Score _______% on each	Pass / Fail / Incomplete
7. Practical Approach interactive workshop	Yes / No	Subjective scores Target Pass	Pass / Fail / Incomplete
8. Flexible bronchoscopy simulation workshop	Yes / No	Target scores 100% BSTAT ______% TBLB/TBNA ____%	Pass / Fail / Incomplete
9. Flexible bronchoscopy patient-based scenario	Yes / No	Target scores 100% BSTAT ______% TBLB/TBNA ____%	Pass / Fail / Incomplete
10. Proctored case bronchoscopy checklist	Yes / No	FB 10-pt Checklist Target 100% Score ______%	Pass / Fail / Incomplete

*When completed, learners are assumed to be able to perform flexible bronchoscopy independently. Programs may still require observation and faculty presence based on training regulations and preferences.

CONGRATULATIONS

You have now completed

The Introduction to Flexible Bronchoscopy Training Manual.

This is an important achievement. We hope this educational experience has been productive and inspiring. In addition to improving your cognitive, affective and experiential knowledge, you have significantly improved your technical skills and your ability to teach others effectively.

Please consider participating in our Faculty Development Programs (Train-the-Trainers) organized by Bronchoscopy International® in collaboration with national and international professional medical societies around the world.

We look forward to receiving your comments regarding our programs

Please do not hesitate to contact your regional organization, or email us at www.bronchoscopy.org

Thank you for participating in **The Bronchoscopy Education Project!**

BRONCHOSCOPY INTERNATIONAL®

Made in the USA
Monee, IL
19 June 2026

54848126R00114